2 WEEKS TO A
YOUNGER

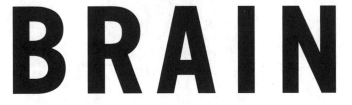

BRAIN

2 WEEKS TO A
YOUNGER

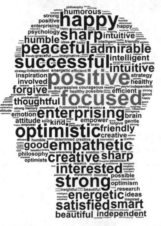

BRAIN

GARY SMALL, MD
AND GIGI VORGAN

Humanix Books

www.humanixbooks.com
Boca Raton, FL, USA

Interior: Ben Davis
Index: Yvette M. Chin

For information, contact:
Humanix Books
P.O. Box 20989
West Palm Beach, FL 33416
USA
www.humanixbooks.com
email: info@humanixbooks.com

Humanix Books is a division of Humanix Publishing, LLC. Its trademark, consisting of the words "Humanix Books" is registered with the US Patent and Trademark Office, and in other countries.

Disclaimer: The information presented in this book is meant to be used for general resource purposes only; it is not intended as specific medical advice for any individual and should not substitute medical advice from a healthcare professional. If you have (or think you may have) a medical problem, speak to your doctor or a healthcare practitioner immediately about your risk and possible treatments. Do not engage in any therapy or treatment without consulting a medical professional.

Printed in the United States of America and the United Kingdom.

ISBN (Hardcover) 978-1-63006-030-5
ISBN (E-book) 978-1-63006-031-2
Library of Congress Control Number: 2014958068

Acknowledgments

W E ARE GRATEFUL TO the many volunteers and patients who participated in the research studies that inspired this book. Thank you to our colleagues and friends who provided their guidance and input, including Susan Bowerman, Howard Chang, and the extraordinary team of doctors, scientists, and staff at UCLA, as well as Diana Jacobs for her drawing on page 152. Special thanks to our dear friend and agent, Sandra Dijkstra, who has nurtured our writing over the years; our publisher, Anthony Ziccardi; our editors, Jon S. Ford and Pamela Pantaleo; and Chris Ruddy, Matthew Kalash, and the entire team at Newsmax Media and Humanix Books. Finally, this book would not have been possible without the love and support of our children, Rachel and Harry, and the rest of our family.

NOTE:

Many stories and examples contained in this book are composite accounts based on the experiences of many individuals and do not represent any one person or group of people. Similarities to any one person or persons are coincidental and unintentional. Readers may wish to talk with their doctor before starting any exercise or diet program.

Contents

	Preface	ix
one	Brain-Boosting Discoveries for a Younger Mind	1
two	Mastering Memory	27
three	Cut Stress to Sharpen Your Mind	51
four	Get Smart with Brain Games	75
five	Food for Thought	105
six	Keep Fit for a Younger Brain	127
seven	Good Friends Make Happy Neurons	151
eight	Mind Your Medicine	171
nine	The 2-Week Younger Brain Program	195
appx 1	Brain Game Websites	237
appx 2	Additional Resources	239
	Bibliography	245
	Index	283

Preface

MISPLACING YOUR KEYS, FORGETTING someone's name at a party, or coming home from the market without the most important item — these are just some of the many common memory slips we all experience from time to time. But such cognitive lapses don't just plague middle-agers and seniors: our UCLA studies indicate that forgetfulness begins much earlier in life. Scientists can detect subtle changes in the brain that coincide with mental decline by the time we reach age 40, and our findings show that people as young as 20 already have memory problems.

Thankfully, the latest research confirms that there is a lot we can do to strengthen our memory and keep our brains young. After three decades of helping thousands of patients improve their memory and mental acuity, I am convinced that our daily lifestyle habits are directly linked to our brain health. My work has shown that it only takes two weeks to form new habits that bolster cognitive abilities and help stave off, or even reverse, brain aging.

In *2 Weeks to a Younger Brain*, the latest brain science is translated into practical strategies and exercises that yield quick and long-lasting benefits. It will not only improve your memory, but it will also strengthen your physical health by reducing your risk for diabetes, heart disease, and stroke.

If you commit only 14 days to my program, I am confident you will reap noticeable results. During that brief period, you will have learned the secrets to keeping your brain young for the rest of your life.

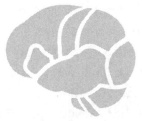

CHAPTER ONE

Brain-Boosting Discoveries for a Younger Mind

"When I was younger, I could remember anything, whether it happened or not."

—*Mark Twain*

HAVE YOU EVER WALKED into a room and forgotten why? What about that awkward feeling of meeting an old friend and blanking on his name? And how many times have you misplaced your glasses or keys?

Most of us laugh about these occasional memory slips, but for some people, it's no joke. Mental lapses become more frequent after age 40, and they can terrify people who worry about dementia. Every misplaced phone or wallet can trigger apprehension: Could this be the beginning of a downward spiral toward Alzheimer's disease?

The good news is that usually these fears are unwarranted. Of course, our brains do gradually age along with our bodies, but we all possess the power to slow, stop, and possibly reverse that brain aging process. The key is learning what causes brain aging and then using effective strategies to beat it. Recent scientific

discoveries show that simply altering some of our everyday behaviors can help keep our minds young and sharp.

We live in a society that equates youth with beauty and power, and some people pursue a younger appearance at any cost.
But even if we could cut 10 or 20 years off our looks, how could
we enjoy it without a sharp, healthy mind? Brain health must be
priority number one, and it turns out that the same strategies
I've developed to keep our brains young also enhance our body's
health and appearance.

Panicked by Forgetfulness

My patient Sharon was a chic and coiffed 62-year-old real estate broker who looked years younger than her age. She wasn't
embarrassed to admit that she visited her plastic surgeon every
four months to get Botox injections. She loved the way he made
the lines around her eyes disappear. Riding down in the elevator from his office recently, she couldn't remember whether
her next stop was the dentist or a meeting with a client. She
searched her purse for her smartphone and panicked when she
couldn't find it. Had she left it at home? Could it be in the car?

As she raced into the parking structure, she suddenly realized
that she hadn't noticed what level she parked on. Sharon hur-
ried past rows and rows of cars, repeatedly pressing the remote
unlock button on her key in hopes of hearing the car beep. After searching two levels, she sat down on a bench to catch her
breath and calm down. This wasn't the first time she'd experienced memory problems, but this episode finally convinced her
to come see me.

Sharon entered my office and took a seat, and I asked how I
could help. She told me that her memory had always been excellent and how much that helped in business. But for the last two
years she'd been having more memory lapses, and they seemed
to be getting worse. I asked her what had been going on in her
life when the memory lapses had begun.

"Well, I had just gone through a messy divorce and decided to have another face-lift. You know, it's good for my job to look young. But since then, I haven't felt quite as sharp. I know it takes weeks, sometimes months to get back to normal after a big procedure, but this is ridiculous. I'm having trouble keeping track of clients, and my sales are slipping. I worry all the time, and frankly, I'm getting depressed about it."

We discussed her feelings of depression for a while, but because general anesthesia can lead to temporary or even chronic memory problems, I wanted to know more about her face-lift two years ago. "How long did the surgery take?" I asked.

"The nurse said I was out for about eight hours."

I was already forming several ideas of what might be contributing to Sharon's complaints. In addition to major surgery, stress from her divorce and job could have been worsening her memory and mood. I reviewed her medical history, medications, and lifestyle habits that might have been affecting her brain health. I described various treatments for depression that might lift her spirits and offered Sharon some tips to improve her recall abilities quickly. At the end of her first session, I recommended that she avoid further elective surgery because of the possible memory effects of surgery requiring general anesthesia.

Sharon laughed. "You're going to have to come up with something better than that, Dr. Small, because I'm getting my eyes done in two weeks."

As we continued to meet over the next few weeks, I was able to convince Sharon to hold off on the surgery. She began her younger brain program and gradually adjusted her lifestyle to include daily exercise, memory training, a healthier diet, and new relaxation techniques to lower her stress. Within a month, Sharon's memory abilities improved, her business picked up, and she felt better than she had in years.

Sharon is not alone. Millions of baby boomers are grappling with their aging and searching for ways to look, think, and feel younger. There's good news: recent studies indicate that our daily habits — what we eat, how much we exercise, the way we interact with others, and how we respond to stress — have a profound impact on our brain aging. Simply making healthy lifestyle choices and practicing easy mental exercises can bolster brain capacity, improve mood, and enhance quality of life.

💡 **DISCOVERY #1:**
Memory does not have to decline with age.

Our UCLA research group has demonstrated a direct link between healthy habits and better memory. In our collaboration with Gallup Poll, we surveyed more than 18,000 people across the United States and found that the more healthy behaviors a person engaged in, the better their recall ability. People who simply practiced one healthy behavior, like eating vegetables or exercising daily, were 21 percent less likely to report memory symptoms than those who reported few if any healthy behaviors. Respondents who engaged in two healthy behaviors had a 45 percent higher chance of a better memory. And those who practiced three healthy habits were 75 percent more likely to have better memory.

The findings of this large-scale survey are consistent with our clinical and brain scan research studies: when individuals engage in a 14-day comprehensive program combining several healthy behaviors — regular physical and mental exercise, a nutritious diet, and stress control — they will alter their brain's neural circuits and help stave off or even halt the effects of brain aging.

💡 **DISCOVERY #2:**
Adopting healthy habits can make your brain younger within two weeks.

What Is a Younger Brain?

I remember a kid in grade school calling me "fat head." At the time, I didn't realize what a compliment that was. A bigger, fatter brain is a healthier and younger brain — one that is packed with sturdy cells. These healthy cells, or neurons, rapidly transfer information through connections called synapses. Tiny neurotransmitters, or packets of information in chemical form, travel across these synapses throughout the brain, helping us think quickly and efficiently. Healthy, young brains have many qualities that keep them functioning at their peak, such as:

- High-performing neurons with strong membranes

- Intact wires or axons connecting those neurons

- Thick myelin — the fatty insulation that surrounds and protects brain wires and speeds up message transmission

- Ample neurotransmitters to convey chemical messages across synapses

- Optimal blood flow providing oxygen and nutrients to neurons

- Minimal abnormal protein deposits that lead to neurodegeneration and brain disease

In general, younger brains are healthier brains, but there are exceptions. For example, a young athlete might suffer a concussion — a traumatic brain injury that can cause confusion, headache, and memory loss. If that athlete is allowed to rest long enough after the injury, his brain will usually recover and return to its healthy, youthful state. But, if the athlete gets right back in the game and adds further stress to his brain, it can prolong his symptoms, and potentially lead to irreversible neurodegeneration or damage.

Unequivocal scientific evidence indicates that getting older is the most significant cause of erosion of cells in our brains and bodies. It's easy to see the common, external, physical evidence of aging: graying hair, wrinkling skin, and expanding waistlines. My patient Sharon's first concern was her appearance — she wanted to maintain her youthful looks and pursued that goal with plastic surgery. Unfortunately, her multiple operations may have worsened her memory and accelerated her brain aging.

 YOU ARE INNATELY SMARTER THAN YOU THINK
I am confident that your brain can unscramble the following sentence quickly:

Teh rihgt psyichal adn mtneal eerxcsie acn ekep oury bairn oyugn.

Meet My Friend What's His Name

I recently ran into a work colleague at the movies, and he paused before introducing me to his wife. I suspected he'd momentarily forgotten my name so I quickly introduced myself as I shook her hand. Perhaps he was distracted by the activity in the busy lobby, or just thrown by seeing me out of context, but that kind of memory slip could have been an indirect clue to his brain age.

Memory slips, or "senior moments," result from the wear and tear of aging on our brains. This wear and tear comes from oxidative stress, inflammation, and other chemical alterations that deteriorate our neurons. Age-related memory declines can be easily assessed with neuropsychological examinations or standardized pencil-and-paper tests.

In 2012, French scientist Archana Singh-Manoux and her colleagues reported results of their 10-year study of cognitive skills in 7,000 middle-aged and older civil servants. They showed that, for most people in their mid-40s, memory and reasoning skills decline by more than three percent per decade. By their mid-60s, that aging process accelerates to greater than seven percent each decade.

One of the most important forms of short-term memory that declines with age is known as *working memory*, which allows us to hold new information in mind long enough to use it, discard it, or send it to long-term memory stores. We use our working memory every day to help us recall where we put things, call phone numbers we've just heard, solve problems, and quickly perform almost any kind of mental work.

In a joint US and UK study, researchers identified the earliest signs of brain aging by measuring *visual* working memory — the ability to keep a visual image in mind for a short period of time. In the study, more than 55,000 volunteers from age eight to 75 looked at various objects for a few moments and then tried to remember their shapes and colors.

The following graph is a plot of the volunteers' memory scores (vertical axis) according to their ages (horizontal axis).

Memory Peaks and Declines with Age

From age eight to 20, memory for colors and shapes improves each year as young brains hone these skills. But after peaking around age 20, this type of memory gradually declines. This pattern suggests that brain aging begins early in adult life and

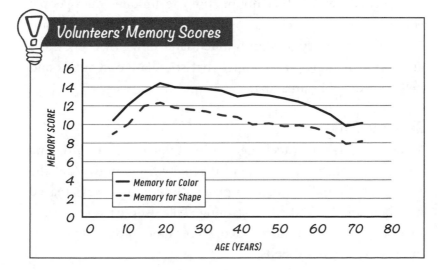

steadily declines so that by age 55, our visual memory abilities may again be equal to those of a 10-year-old.

QUICK BRAIN-BUIDLING TEASER:
Two cab drivers are going the wrong way on a one-way street. A policeman sees them and doesn't give them a ticket. Can you think of a plausible explanation? *(Answer at the end of chapter.)*

This decline in memory for colors and shapes could explain why even young adults often forget where they put things like their phones or wallets. Although our most recent UCLA studies document memory complaints for people as young as age 18, most of us don't notice or worry about memory loss until middle age. One explanation is that by age 40, additional types of memory-slips kick in. At that point, our ability to remember names and faces becomes the most common memory complaint. People in their 40s also begin having difficulty recalling certain words and details — the information just doesn't roll off the tip of their tongue as easily as it used to, even though they are sure they know it.

The good news is that my memory techniques help people compensate for age-related cognitive declines, so they may not experience memory loss until much later in life, if ever. There are also many new technologies that stimulate our minds and help slow down brain aging.

Reset the Clock

When my son was a teenager, I used to give him a hard time about how much time he spent playing video games. And the few times I actually agreed to play with him, he always teased me about my limited video-gaming skills. I didn't realize then that playing some of those video games more often might have improved my mental skills.

DISCOVERY #3
Some video games can subtract decades from your brain age.

Scientists have revealed that simply playing certain video games less than 30 minutes each day can greatly enhance multitasking skills. Scientists at the University of California, San Francisco, found that the brain performance of a 70-year-old can be transformed into that of a 20-year-old by simply playing a video game that trains drivers to ignore distractions. Whether you train your brain best by playing a video game, attending a lecture, or following a written program, you have the power to bolster your neural circuits and enhance your brain efficiency, resulting in a younger brain.

The benefits of brain training on memory skills can be quick and remarkable. In my lectures, I often teach the audience a few memory exercises to improve their recall skills within minutes. I show them how focusing on new information and putting it into a meaningful framework will make it memorable.

Prove it to yourself by trying to remember the words below. Instead of using rote memorization, however, try creating a story that uses the words. Because the words are unrelated, the story you create may sound silly, but that actually makes it easier to remember. The words in your story don't have to appear in this order.

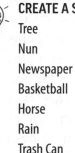

CREATE A STORY USING THE WORDS BELOW:
Tree
Nun
Newspaper
Basketball
Horse
Rain
Trash Can

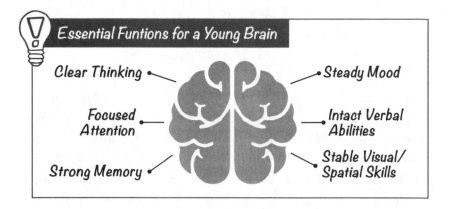

One story example could be: A *nun* riding a *horse* stops under a *tree* because it's starting to *rain*. She covers her head with a *newspaper* that gets all wet, so she rolls it up and tosses it like a *basketball* into a *trash can*.

Although people tend to complain most about their memory as they age, it's not the only mental skill that may decline. Luckily, training our memory also boosts our attention, language, and problem-solving abilities. Paying attention is critical to learning and recall because when we are distracted, we don't always absorb the new information we may wish to remember later. A strong memory is vital for clear thinking and reasoning, as well as navigating our three-dimensional world (visual-spatial skills). Strengthening these mental functions helps keep our brains young.

A Window into the Brain

My first job in high school was assisting a radiologist at a local community hospital. I helped develop X-rays in the darkroom and escorted patients by wheelchair from their rooms to the radiology department and back. The high-tech equipment that let doctors peer inside the body and the brain fascinated me — up until then I thought only superheroes had X-ray vision.

But we really weren't seeing much of the brain with those early X-rays. Instead, we saw pictures of boney structures like the skull that surrounds and protects the delicate brain tissue.

Over the next few decades, remarkable technological advances in brain imaging methods began to yield exquisite ways to see the details of what's going on in people's heads. These developments provided newer tools such as magnetic resonance imaging (MRI) and positron-emission tomography (PET), which now allow scientists to peek into the living brain and detect changes that are occurring in real time — a virtual window into the brain.

DISCOVERY #4
Memory training can erase senior moments from your
brain scan.

MRI scans are commonly used in clinical settings to view the brain's structure; they allow for detection of tumors, strokes (dead brain cells), or atrophy (brain shrinkage). Functional MRI can show brain activity from moment to moment. This powerful scanning method allows neuroscientists to observe and measure neural circuits that are working harder to compensate for age-associated memory decline — we can actually see our senior moments. After practicing simple memory exercises for

Einstein's Brain

When Albert Einstein died in 1955, his heirs donated his brain to science, and researchers have been studying it ever since. A recent analysis measured the size of different areas of his brain. As you might have guessed, some of Professor Einstein's important brain regions were much larger compared to those of an average person. A thick band of nerve fibers separating the left and right sides of his brain (known as the corpus callosum) was particularly hefty. These fibers transmit information between the brain's left and right hemispheres, and this thicker corpus callosum could explain Einstein's superior intellectual capacity. Also, his frontal lobe was larger than normal. There is good news for those of us who are not Einsteins: mental and physical exercise not only increase brain mass, they boost memory and cognitive abilities too.

a brief period, our brains become more proficient. A repeat MRI scan will document improved brain efficiency, and those previously observed senior moments no longer appear in the scan.

Many of our UCLA studies have confirmed the close link between the outward manifestations of brain health (e.g., memory ability, language skills) and actual biological brain aging that shows up on MRI and PET scans. People who perform better on pencil-and-paper memory tests actually have bigger brains that function better. My team's research has shown that an individual's subjective memory rating, or their own awareness of their memory changes, reflects underlying biological changes in their brain structure. If you *feel* like you are losing your memory, it can often be documented in a brain scan.

PET scanning shows the details of brain structure as well as brain function. A PET scanner works like a Geiger counter because it measures radioactivity. The doctor injects the patient with a tiny amount of radioactive chemical marker that travels through the blood system into the brain, allowing the PET scanner to measure how much chemical is accumulating in different brain regions. Depending on the type of chemical the doctor injects, different biological changes can be detected.

When PET imaging was first introduced to the medical world, we were awed by the colorful images — it was like seeing color television for the first time. In PET scans, brain areas that are active light up in bright reds, oranges, and yellows. The most common chemical marker used with PET is a form of glucose (sugar) — the brain's main energy source. Numerous PET scan investigations have shown that younger brains utilize more sugar. You can see the warm colors that indicate the brain cells are firing up in a normal and active way, particularly in the areas that control memory, reasoning, and other cognitive skills.

PET studies also show that with aging, these same brain regions gradually lose their ability to burn sugar efficiently, indicating decline in brain function. The scans show this subtle decline in healthy people beginning in their 40s, approximately the same age when neuropsychologists can begin to detect brain aging with pencil-and-paper tests.

People whose PET scan shows lower activity on the left side of the brain, which controls language skills, have a harder time performing verbal memory tests. Those whose scans show lower activity on the right side of the brain, which controls visual and spatial abilities, struggle more with reading maps and recalling three-dimensional images. If you're left-handed, the functions of your right and left brain are reversed.

After performing hundreds of PET studies using the conventional sugar marker, our UCLA research team wanted to take the technology a step further. A small group of us began to look for more precise ways to peer inside the brain, and we synthesized a new chemical marker (FDDNP) that allowed PET scanners to measure the most definitive signs of brain aging — abnormal protein deposits known as amyloid plaques and tau tangles. These plaques and tangles are the physical evidence of Alzheimer's disease and begin to accumulate gradually in the brain decades before symptoms of the disease emerge. The scans of patients with cognitive losses typical of Alzheimer's dementia show significantly elevated FDDNP-PET signals in brain areas that control memory, thinking, and other cognitive abilities. These special PET scans reveal subtle signals of abnormal protein buildup in people with only very mild memory complaints.

When someone has Alzheimer's disease, some brain regions are ravaged while others are spared. Autopsy studies after the deaths of patients with Alzheimer's disease show plaques and tangles in the same brain areas that FDDNP-PET scans can pick up in living patients.

Three Stages of Brain Aging

Our brain scan studies have detailed the three major stages of brain aging: normal aging, mild cognitive impairment, and dementia. In our 40s or sometimes younger, we begin to notice mild forgetfulness that has minimal impact on our daily lives. This stage is termed *normal aging*. If we fail to protect our brains from the aging process, normal aging can transition to mild cognitive impairment. Although we then notice more everyday memory difficulties, we can still compensate for them and live independently. If that compensation ability breaks down, people begin to suffer from dementia, and the most common form of dementia is Alzheimer's.

If normal brain aging transitions to mild cognitive impairment, FDDNP-PET scans begin to show some accumulation of plaques and tangles in areas that control memory, particularly in the hippocampus (temporal lobe). If brain aging continues to advance toward dementia, abnormalities show up in regions that regulate language (Broca's area), reasoning and planning skills (frontal lobe), memory and emotion (temporal lobe), and perception and personality (parietal lobe). However, the sensorimotor strip (sensation and movement), the visual cortex (sight), and the cerebellum (balance) remain relatively stable — even in patients with Alzheimer's dementia.

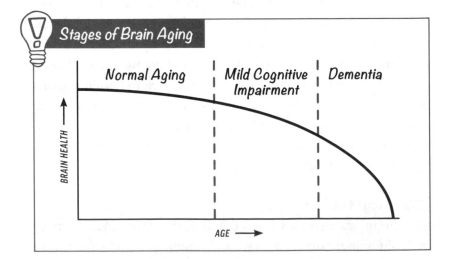

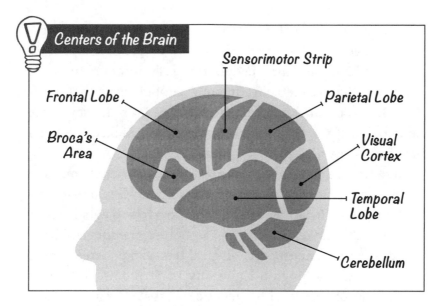

Centers of the Brain

Sensorimotor Strip

Frontal Lobe

Parietal Lobe

Broca's Area

Visual Cortex

Temporal Lobe

Cerebellum

Don't Just Blame Your Genes

When I was a kid, I was friends with identical twins, Stuart and Steve. I used to have a hard time telling them apart back then. They would play tricks on me where Steve would pretend he was Stuart and vice versa. But when I got to know them better, I could tell who was who because of their different personalities. I got along best with Steve — we played basketball together and joked around a lot. Stuart was more serious and sensitive — he'd often take things the wrong way and get insulted. When I ran into them again years later, they were very different. Stuart was overweight, divorced, and smoked heavily. Steve appeared athletic and healthy and told me he was married with three children.

My childhood experience was consistent with research showing that even in identical twins, different qualities and habits emerge as a result of their environment and life experiences. However, some behaviors and traits are surprisingly driven by inheritance.

In the late 1970s and early 1980s, investigators at the University of Minnesota studied identical adult twins that were reared apart. They found remarkable similarities in many

measures of personality, personal interests, and tempera-
ment, suggesting that genetics has a much greater impact on
taste and character than people realized. Some of the twin
pairs, who hadn't met since infancy, actually gave their children the exact same name or drove the exact same car in the
same color. If the twins smoked, they often picked the same
brand of cigarette.

Genetics are certainly not the whole story when it comes to
brain aging. Our UCLA research shows that when one identical twin lives a healthier lifestyle (e.g., exercises, eats healthy,
and doesn't smoke), that twin has better memory abilities,
higher scores on neuropsychological tests, and a larger brain.
Scientists at Washington University in St. Louis found that
brain scans of people with a genetic risk for Alzheimer's show
less evidence of the disease in their brains if they exercise
regularly.

DISCOVERY #5:
Lifestyle habits affect your brain more than your genes do.

The large-scale longitudinal MacArthur Study defined successful aging as maintaining both cognitive and physical health.
That landmark study showed that for the average individual,
nongenetic factors contribute more to successful aging than
the DNA we inherit. Scientists have since uncovered several of
these *non*genetic factors, like lifestyle choices and environmental influences that are often under our control.

When I first began researching the neuroscience of aging,
doctors hadn't yet discovered any genes that contributed to dementia, but we did know that people with a family history of
Alzheimer's have a higher risk of developing it themselves. In
order to understand the genetic connection, I collaborated with
scientists from Duke University to study families with several
affected relatives. These collaborations led to the discovery of

the first major gene known to influence the risk for Alzheimer's disease: apolipoprotein E, or APOE.

Detailing the genetics was tricky because you don't know who will develop Alzheimer's disease until late in life. Today, we hear a lot more about Alzheimer's because people are living longer — life expectancy has nearly doubled during the past century, and age is the greatest risk factor for cognitive decline. Most people are terrified of developing dementia, defined as cognitive decline that leaves the patient dependent on others. Alzheimer's disease accounts for nearly two-thirds of all dementias, and scientists are more motivated than ever to unravel its genetics, because knowing what causes an illness often leads to better treatments and possibly a cure.

Everybody carries one of the three forms, or alleles, of the APOE gene in their DNA, but only one of them — the APOE-4 allele — heightens the risk for Alzheimer's disease. One out of every five people is a carrier of APOE-4, but not all APOE-4 carriers develop the disease, while others who do not have APOE-4 do get Alzheimer's. Therefore, the gene alone does not provide enough information to be a predictive test. However, when we combine someone's brain scan and their genetic data, we get a more precise picture of their brain health. In fact, it's now possible to detect subtle evidence of brain aging and Alzheimer's disease decades before an individual actually develops symptoms.

The other forms of the gene, APOE-2 and APOE-3, work to keep the brain young, but the mechanism is not clear. We do know that the proteins produced by all forms of APOE transport cholesterol in the blood. Since some forms of cholesterol like LDL (bad cholesterol) are unhealthy for the brain, it's possible that the three forms of APOE affect the brain differently due to the way they convey cholesterol.

Since we initially discovered APOE, scientists have found other genes that may help keep the brain young. BDNF (short

Test Your Knowledge

Answer the following multiple choice question:
People who complete a college education:

    A. Have a higher risk for developing Alzheimer's disease

    B. Have a lower risk for developing Alzheimer's disease

    C. Are more arrogant than non-graduates

    D. None of the above

Correct Answer

    B. Scientists attribute the association between education and lower Alzheimer's risk to the mental stimulation that education provides. But it could also be a result of the fact that educated people are more likely to be aware that habits, like exercising and not smoking, are good for their health.

for *brain-derived neurotrophic factor*) is a gene that stimulates brain cell growth and strengthens the connections between neurons. Another gene associated with a lower Alzheimer's risk, TREM2, interacts with the body's inflammatory system and may control age-related inflammation by staving off mental and physical aging.

Mental stimulation, physical exercise, diet, and other healthy lifestyle habits have a stronger impact on keeping our brains young than genetics. We demonstrated this impact when we studied the effects of educational achievement on brain function. After performing PET scans on volunteers of various ages, we compared the results of those with and without a college degree. College graduates ranging from their 20s to their 50s displayed higher activity in brain memory regions than people who had not graduated from college. Getting a college degree actually affected brain function more than possessing the good APOE-2 or APOE-3 gene allele. Of course, a healthy genetic roll of the dice may increase the likelihood of someone attending college, but once there, the enriched educational environment further boosts brain health and keeps neurons active and resilient, even decades later.

Sex, Drugs, and Rock and Roll

Not long ago, Paul McCartney admitted to forgetting some of the lyrics to his early Beatles songs. I imagined him singing, "She loves you, wow, wow, wow . . ." McCartney's disclosure probably made a lot of baby boomers feel better about forgetting some of the lyrics to their own favorite oldies.

Music has a powerful effect on the brain. Recent studies indicate that when we listen to music we enjoy, it improves both our mood and our memory. Even people with mild cognitive impairment can increase their learning and recall abilities after just a week of listening to their favorite tunes.

Music activates the brain's dopamine reward system as well as its emotional control center, the amygdala (*ah-mig-de-lah*) — an almond-shaped knob of tissue deep in the center of the brain. When we enjoy music, our brain gets flooded with the feel-good dopamine neurotransmitter.

DISCOVERY #6
Listening to music can improve your mental abilities.

Functional MRI studies show that our early exposure to different types of music will shape our musical preferences. If you grew up listening to rock and roll, chances are you prefer the Rolling Stones over Mozart. Listening to a favorite song or classical piece often sparks chemical reactions in our brains that lift or lower our mood, depending on how we felt when we first connected with the music.

Musical memories can be strong emotional triggers. If you fell in love at a time when you were enjoying a particular song, listening to that song years later probably elicits warm and romantic memories. If you were heartbroken at a time when a particular song was popular, hearing that tune may make you feel sad.

The 1960s and '70s was a time when many baby boomers listened to rock and roll while experimenting with recreational drugs. With the nearly 80 million boomers now beginning to turn 65 — the age when their risk for Alzheimer's increases to 10 percent — many wonder whether their drug use back in the day may have contributed to their current age-related memory complaints.

Marijuana was the most frequently used recreational drug at that time, and chronic use has been shown to impair memory and attention. The good news is that any potentially harmful effects of marijuana on brain function appear to diminish after people stop or cut back on their use of the drug. But the cognitive effects of marijuana vary depending upon the strain of the cannabis. The main active ingredient in marijuana, tetrahydrocannabinol (THC), causes the euphoria that many users enjoy, while a second chemical, cannabidiol, has a calming effect. Investigators at the University of London found that marijuana low in cannabidiol impairs recall during intoxication, whereas strains of the drug that are high in cannabidiol do not seem to impair cognition.

Some people report that using marijuana enhances their sexual enjoyment. However, making love, with or without pot, appears to have its own positive effect on brain health.

DISCOVERY #7
A healthy sex life is good for your brain.

Dr. Benedetta Leuner and associates at Princeton University and Claremont Colleges found that daily sexual activity in laboratory animals reduced stress, stimulated growth of new memory cells in the brain, and strengthened connections between those cells. In human studies, more frequent sexual activity in men has been associated with longer life expectancy. This may result from the release of the hormone DHEA during orgasm, which lowers the risk for a heart attack. Orgasm also reduces tension and helps both men and women sleep better, in part through the release of endorphins and other hormones.

Remaining sexually active also improves the body's immune system — its ability to fight off infections. In a study of college students, those engaging in sexual activity once or twice a week had a 30 percent higher immunoglobulin A level compared to students who were sexually abstinent. Immunoglobulin A is one of our most important antibodies that protects us from infectious diseases.

You don't have to be intimate with someone for your brain to benefit from social interactions with them. Just having an engaging discussion boosts cognitive health. Psychologists at the University of Michigan found that even a brief but stimulating conversation will increase memory performance and mental speed. And if you chat with an empathic friend about a troubling issue, that interaction can lower your stress levels and further protect your brain neurons.

DISCOVERY #8
A 10-minute conversation increases mental acuity.

The Mind's Power over the Body

Our minds also have a tremendous impact on our physical well-being. Stress, anxiety, and fear can aggravate a variety of physical illnesses, including asthma, heart disease, ulcerative colitis, and hypertension.

One example of the mind's power over the body is when someone's face turns red from feelings of embarrassment or anger. Our emotional states lead to a cascade of chemical reactions in our bodies. Acute or chronic stress causes the adrenal glands to secrete stress hormones like cortisol, which can harm the heart, stomach, and brain. Chronic elevations in cortisol impair cognition and actually shrink some of the brain's important memory centers. People prone to stress have a greater risk for developing Alzheimer's disease, which is the most common result of brain aging.

DISCOVERY #9
Reducing chronic stress improves brain function.

Fortunately, positive emotions can protect our brain's neural circuitry. Good feelings — including love, excitement, and joy — can bring about chemical changes that strengthen physical health. Numerous studies have linked positive emotional states to lower rates of physical illness and symptoms, as well as a higher tolerance of pain. Happiness and pleasure can increase the levels of many feel-good neurotransmitters that circulate throughout the brain and the body, such as dopamine, serotonin, and adrenaline.

Dr. Helen Fisher and colleagues at Stony Brook University in New York used functional MRI scans to identify the brain regions that get activated when people are in love. Her group showed that brain scans of romantic partners light up when they think about each other. The most active brain regions are those that produce the brain chemicals associated with pleasure.

I have seen the powerful effect the mind has on the body and the strong influence the body has on the mind in my own practice. I treated a patient who was an avid swimmer. He began swimming to relieve his lower back pain, but over the years his daily swim not only helped control his back pain, he came to believe he needed it to maintain his energy level and positive frame of mind — he craved the endorphin mood-lift of his water workouts. When he later reinjured his back, his orthopedist ordered strict bed rest. After two weeks of lying around, his back pain did gradually improve, but he became depressed. When he was finally able to swim again, his depression lifted almost immediately.

DISCOVERY #10
A healthy body boosts brainpower.

Whenever I evaluate a patient for a mental symptom, I first explore any possible physical or medical issues that could be causing symptoms of depression, anxiety, or dementia. Sometimes a thyroid imbalance, anemia, heart condition, or even an upper respiratory infection can lead to symptoms of anxiety, depression, or dementia. These kinds of mind and body interactions are not only essential to consider for an accurate diagnosis, but they play an important role in shaping practical strategies for improving and maintaining brain health.

Rewiring Your Brain for Youth

Although my patient Sharon, the real estate broker, consulted me out of concern for her memory, she was also very concerned about maintaining a young appearance. Her pursuit of youth had led to multiple elective surgeries and repeated exposures to anesthesia, which can accelerate brain aging. I was eventually able to convince Sharon to reevaluate her priorities and put her brain health ahead of her physical appearance. When she truly realized she had the ability to improve her memory, she became motivated to make healthy lifestyle changes and began my program to keep her brain young.

Sharon postponed all further elective surgeries and started doing daily fitness workouts that got her heart pumping more oxygen and nutrients to her hungry neurons. I taught her some basic memory methods to help her overcome her senior moments, so she no longer worried about forgetting where she parked her car. It also became easier for her to remember her clients' names and the details of their transactions. Sharon began meditating, which helped her cope with the daily stress of her job, and she noticed a marked lift in her mood. She also

enriched her diet with brain-healthy omega-3 fats from fish and
nuts, as well as antioxidant fruits and vegetables. After just one
week on her program, Sharon reported better recall skills, and
when I reassessed her after a month, she showed significant improvements in both her verbal and visual memory scores.

 DID YOU KNOW?
Your brain uses approximately 20 percent of all the oxygen and
nutrients in your entire body.

Protect Your Head

Throughout life, a variety of illnesses and accidents can compromise neural circuitry and accelerate brain aging, including head trauma, surgery, elevated blood pressure, and small
strokes. When severe, these incidents cause permanent damage, but often such brain injuries are temporary, especially
when people protect their brains from further damage. Healthy
brains are able to compensate for many injuries and even grow
new, sturdy cells.

Dr. Fred Gage of the Salk Institute in La Jolla, California, and
other scientists have shown that new nerve growth, or neurogenesis, is possible in adult brains. Our UCLA research has
demonstrated that brain-training exercises and healthy lifestyle
choices can activate the brain's neural circuits and make them

Madame Jeanne Calment of France

One of the oldest documented individuals was Madame Jeanne Calment, who lived
to 122 years. She exercised regularly, ate a brain-healthy diet, remained active
mentally, and had no signs of dementia throughout her long life. Her sharp mental
acuity was apparent in some of her business transactions. At the age of 94, she sold
her apartment to an entrepreneur who agreed to let her remain in the flat rent-free
for the rest of her life. The entrepreneur died 10 years later, and Madame Calment
continued to live rent-free for another 28 years.

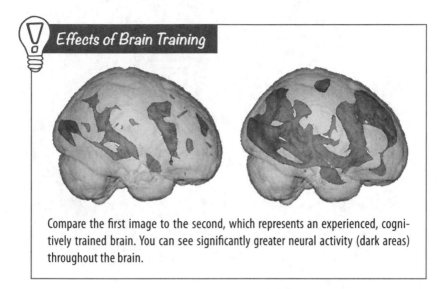

Effects of Brain Training

Compare the first image to the second, which represents an experienced, cognitively trained brain. You can see significantly greater neural activity (dark areas) throughout the brain.

more efficient. The above functional MRI scans show how an untrained brain appears when engaged in a mental challenge.

Living Longer and Sharper

By keeping our brains young, we can expect more enjoyment in our later years. Advances in medical technology have extended the average life expectancy in the United States and other developed countries from 46 years for someone born in 1900 to 78 years for someone born today. Many scientists now estimate that the average human life span may eventually approach 120 years.

The evidence is clear: a younger brain is a better brain. As you read through the following chapters, you will learn strategies to help you to take control over your own brain aging. With practice, these strategies will strengthen your neural circuits, and you will soon notice improved memory and mental clarity.

ANSWER TO BRAIN-BUILDING TEASER
PAGE 8: Two cab drivers.
    The cab drivers are *walking* the wrong way on a one-way street.

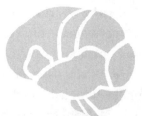

CHAPTER TWO

Mastering Memory

"Right now I'm having amnesia and déjà vu at the
same time. I think I've forgotten this before."
—*Steven Wright*

F OR MANY YEARS I have flown back and forth from Los Angeles to Washington, DC, to review research grants for the
National Institutes of Health. Returning from a particularly
intense meeting where I had pored over hundreds of pages
of scientific proposals, I stopped at an airport bookshop to
buy a paperback to read on the flight. I craved some engaging
fiction to help me escape all the technical jargon I had been
immersed in.

As I browsed the shelves, a Ken Follett novel piqued my interest. I had read several of his books, and although the characters in his stories tended to have a familiarity to them, there
were always twists and turns that drew me in. I skimmed the
synopsis on the back of the book. It was a thriller involving po-
litical intrigue, catching terrorists, and a love triangle — ingredients that could help ease my mental fatigue.

On my flight, I got about 25 pages into the book when I had a Ken Follett déjà vu experience — the scene was *too* familiar. I realized I had read the book about five years earlier. I supposed that the redesigned cover of the paperback version had tricked me into buying it again. I felt foolish — why hadn't I recalled that I had already read the book from the first few pages or even the synopsis on the back?

Photographic Memory

Usually memory doesn't work that way. Unless memories have special meaning to us, our brains seldom store them for more than a brief time. There are, however, a very small number of individuals who do remember every detail of their past experiences. These people possess highly superior autobiographical memory, or hyperthymesia — what many people refer to as a photographic memory. They have an unusual ability to recall specific personal events and extremely trivial details of their lives.

Dr. James McGaugh and colleagues at the University of California, Irvine, reported a case of a woman with this syndrome who had "nonstop, uncontrollable, and automatic" memory abilities. If you gave her a date, she could tell you exactly what she wore, ate, or did on that day. She remembered trivial details of insignificant experiences just as much as she recalled major events. Most of us remember what we were doing the day we learned John Kennedy or John Lennon was shot, but do we recall what we were doing the day before? Usually not.

The brain wiring of individuals with such extraordinary autobiographical memory likely differs from 99 percent of the population. Using MRI and PET scanning, researchers have found that their brains have better connections in regions that transmit information between the temporal and frontal lobes. This finding backs up other studies indicating that when this pathway is injured, autobiographical memory is impaired.

McGaugh speculates that people with this type of superior autobiographical memory are inundated with mental stimuli and not able to discern what information is important to remember and what is not. To them, all memories are created equal.

Being a hyperthymestic individual might have its advantages if you're taking an SAT test or preparing for the bar exam, but in everyday life it may not offer much practical benefit. In fact, many of these individuals have trouble forgetting unpleasant memories and suffer from obsessive-compulsive symptoms, such as hoarding or mysophobia (fear of germs), as well as the need to categorize and control every aspect of their lives. It must be exhausting for them.

Memory: The Long and Short of It

Fortunately our brains have adapted so that everyday memory function is practical and useful. Our brains are programmed to see the big picture from moment to moment. We only tend to remember details that are meaningful to us and ignore the trivia. This process filters out a lot of minutiae that are not useful. I remembered some of the key plot points of the Follett novel, as well as the personalities of the major characters, but I had forgotten the title and the general aspects of the story. Perhaps if I had spotted the original cover of the hardback I read, I might have recognized the novel, but the new cover tricked my brain into forgetting that I had read it.

Every day our brains are bombarded with sensory input, but they are hardwired to pick and choose what input is important and meaningful so we can recall it later. Without that capacity, our brains would constantly be overwhelmed sorting through a vast amount of trivia to make sense of it all.

Neuropsychologists have a term for that flow of trivia: sensory memories. At every moment in our wakeful state, our senses flood our brains with a multitude of sensory memories. Our neural circuits create brief records of these events, but very few

of them make it into our long-term memory storage to be re-
tained and retrieved later.

I was aware of this phenomenon as I was drifting off to sleep
the other night; I began to notice the different sounds I heard
in my bedroom. This can actually be a calming mental exercise
that forces our minds to focus and relax. My mind drifted from
one sound to another:

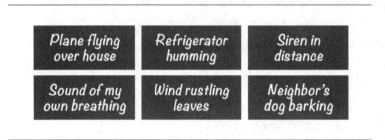

Paying attention to these six sensory memories actually altered my brain chemistry so that these fleeting sensory memories now transformed into short-term memories. Because I
don't usually need nor try to memorize these types of short-
term memories, they never became long-term memories — the
next day, week, or year, I probably wouldn't recall the details of
most of this experience at all.

That night, however, I stopped focusing on most of the passing sensory memories because one of the sounds took center
stage in my mind — my neighbor's dog barking. That same dog
had been barking ferociously for weeks and disturbing everyone
in the neighborhood. The sound meant something to me and
stirred up feelings of resentment. I started thinking about ways
to deal with this nuisance and, as a result, had trouble drifting
off to sleep. This one noise was pushing the other sounds into
the background.

Although my neighbor's dog eventually stopped barking, my
feelings about it lingered on. My experience offers a clue to how
our built-in mental circuits work to form strong new memories.

In this case, my emotions and the ongoing situation next door made the memory meaningful and thus hard to forget. When something is meaningful, it becomes memorable.

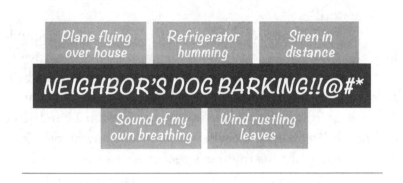

How Did I Get to Work?

For something to become memorable, it first has to catch our attention. Many people today live busy lifestyles — they rush from place to place and they are bombarded by so many sensory memories that their minds tend to be more distracted than focused. New technologies — computers, smartphones, tablets, and other devices — are everywhere. They help us store information and provide an external memory storage source to augment our biological memories, but we can become so preoccupied with them that we fail to focus our attention on learning new information that might be important for us to remember.

Not long ago, Stephen, a 64-year-old history professor, consulted with me because of his gradually declining memory. He said that his research and lectures were fine, but he had trouble remembering things like his weekend errands or the name of a movie he had just seen. I asked him when he first started noticing his memory symptoms, and he said they began about a year ago after his 85-year-old mother was diagnosed with Alzheimer's disease. He finally called me because of an incident that happened the week before.

"I was preparing for my freshman European History class, and my teaching assistant came in a little late, complaining about how bad the traffic was. It occurred to me that I hadn't noticed the traffic. In fact, I had absolutely no recall at all of my drive to work."

It's not uncommon for people to fail to notice their surroundings and experiences of routine daily events like their drive to and from work. Most people are on automatic pilot during these activities and not paying much attention. They may be hunting through radio stations in their car or engrossed in a hands-free phone call. Stephen's concerns were typical of many people in his age group, and his mother's recent Alzheimer's diagnosis likely increased his awareness of his normal age-related memory decline. I predicted it would be relatively easy to help Stephen improve his age-related memory symptoms using some easy memory techniques.

Expert memory champions have devised lots of complicated mnemonic methods to help them remember impressive amounts of information — full pages from phone books or names of hundreds of people in an audience. But many ordinary people find those strategies difficult to learn and not very practical.

My approach involves simple, easy-to-use techniques to overcome everyday memory complaints like forgetting names and where we put things. In fact, you can dramatically eliminate much of your everyday forgetfulness by using my two basic memory methods: FOCUS and FRAME.

FOCUS: Pay Attention to What You Want to Remember

Memory has two essential components: learning and recall. When our memory works, we allow new information into our brain cells and are able to retrieve and recall those memories later. The main reason we forget information such as names or where we put things is that we're not *FOCUSing* our attention to begin with. My first basic memory method, FOCUS, will improve your attention and learning abilities so you can rapidly transfer new information into your memory stores, or what neuropsychologists call *encoding*.

During Stephen's daily commute to work, his mind often wandered; he thought about his schedule for the day, things he wanted to do on the weekend, and numerous other random reflections. He was so familiar with his commute that he did not need to pay much attention and he didn't notice many details of his environment on the way. Of course, if a car stopped short in

Photo Recall

Try this exercise for yourself. Study the photograph below for 30 seconds, noting as much detail as possible; then, cover the photo and see if you can answer the questions below.

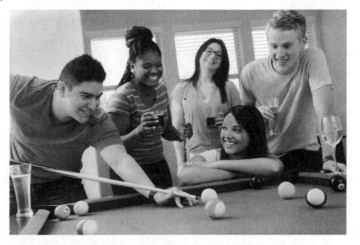

- How many people are in the photo? How many are women?
- How many billiard balls are on the table?
- How many people are holding glasses?
- Was anyone wearing a striped top?
- How many windows were there? Drapes or shades?
- Was everybody standing?

front of him or a pedestrian suddenly dashed into the street, he would immediately slam on his brakes and focus his attention to avoid an accident. He had years of driving experience so that these responses were automatic, and he really had no reason to want to remember other unremarkable things going on around him during the drive.

After checking to make sure that Stephen did not have any serious memory deficits that might indicate Alzheimer's or some other dementia, I began working with him to improve his memory abilities. I started by teaching him a few simple mental exercises to improve his focus and attention span. I had him study a photograph for 30 seconds and concentrate on as many details as possible. He then closed his eyes, and I asked him questions to see how much detail he could recall.

With practice, your ability to recall details will improve. This kind of exercise trains your concentration abilities and helps you focus your attention on new information from moment to

Practice Your Mental Focus Skills

Many people find that when they enhance their ability to pay attention, their recall skills improve almost immediately. Try these easy exercises and see how well you do.

As you watch a movie or TV show, make a conscious effort to pay attention to particular details. You can choose to focus your attention on props, hairdos, wardrobe, or whatever you like. Test yourself the next day to see how much detail you recall. If you saw the show with a friend or your spouse, dazzle them with your attention skills by casually mentioning the grand piano in the room where the butler dropped the tray.

The next time you have a conversation with someone, try to pay particular attention to what that person is saying. Make a mental note of some small detail, particularly one that you think the person might not expect you to remember — it could be where she plans to have dinner that night or what time she has to go to the dentist. See if you remember the detail the next day. If so, give that person a call or send her a text to ask how it went. Mastering this exercise not only boosts your memory ability, but also improves your social skills and can make you more popular.

moment. Although such details may seem trivial, this skill is essential for training your mind to encode new memories.

FRAME: Make New Information Meaningful and Memorable

A few years ago, I had a meeting with a small publishing company on the East Coast. I was introduced to a dozen or so junior editors and assistants while we all waited for the senior editor to arrive. As we made small talk about the weather and sports, I used my memory methods to learn everyone's name. I met a *Diane*, whose purple-highlighted hair must have been *dyed*. *Jack* was in great physical shape so I imagined him doing jumping *jacks*. I envisioned *Suzie* at the dinner table spinning a lazy *Susan*. *Jacob's* beard reminded me of the biblical character *Jacob*. In this way all of their names and faces meant something to me so I could remember them.

When the senior editor came in and asked if I'd met everyone, I responded by naming everybody in the room. He was impressed and asked how I did it. I explained my FOCUS and FRAME method. When I meet someone new, I simply FOCUS my attention on their name and face and FRAME that information together with imaginary pictures I create in my mind. If I meet someone named Joe, I FOCUS my attention and FRAME his name and face with an image of him drinking a cup of *joe* (coffee).

Imagine the brain's memory system as a big filing cabinet. When we FOCUS, we identify the specific information or image that we want to file away for later. But that information needs a FRAME, or folder, that tells us *where* to file it in the cabinet so that we are able to remember its location if we need it. Unfortunately, our neural circuits don't sort information in alphabetical order or use the Dewey decimal system as an organizing tool. We must draw upon our own imagination and ingenuity to file those memories away systematically so we can retrieve them when we want to.

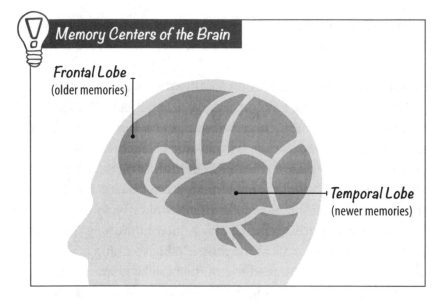

I find that FOCUS and FRAME is the most effective method for remembering names and faces, as well as the easiest. This technique utilizes the brain's hippocampus — the structure underneath the temples in the temporal lobe, where new memories are encoded. (Head trauma that causes damage to the hippocampus or temporal lobe can result in anterograde amnesia, a condition that makes it impossible to form new memories.) The brain's frontal lobe, or thinking brain, then collaborates with the temporal lobe to analyze new information and decide whether it is worth remembering. If the new information proves worthy, it gets consolidated and enters long-term memory storage.

Drs. Christine Smith and Larry Squire at the University of California, San Diego, recently performed functional MRI experiments to pinpoint where long-term memories are stored in the brain. Their findings indicate that our memories begin in the temporal lobe and travel through a neural information highway that moves toward the frontal lobe over time. They also found that the age of a particular memory determines its actual location in the brain. Structures deep beneath the temples in the temporal lobe (the hippocampus and the brain's emotional center, the amygdala) are often less involved with older memories. It's the frontal lobe that stores and manages our very long-term memories.

Seeing Is Remembering

We all know the proverb "Seeing is believing." People often don't accept something as true until they have seen it with their own eyes. When it comes to learning and recall, seeing is remembering, too.

The evolution of our ancient ancestors' brains favored visual acuity because of the survival advantage it provided. If early

---

Practice Linking Unrelated Words

An effective way to strengthen your framing skills is to practice linking up unrelated words. Neuropsychologists often use this approach to test a person's short-term memory abilities. The psychologist shows the patient a list of unrelated word pairs and, after a pause, presents the first word of each pair as the patient tries to recall the second word of the pair.

Here is an example of such a word pair:

Apple — Sponge

If this were a related word pair, like apple-tree, it would be easy for me to see apples growing on a tree, but the above pair is not so obvious. With a little imagination, though, I can visualize myself using a sponge to wash an apple.

Now you practice with the following word pairs:

Window — Teddy Bear
Volcano — Rubber Band
Plate — Cloud
Light Bulb — Movie Star

I came up with several answers, and perhaps yours were similar. I saw a teddy bear displayed in a shop window. I used a huge rubber band to squeeze the tip of a volcano so it would not erupt. I threw a plate like a Frisbee up into a cloud. My movie star accepted her Academy Award wearing a gorgeous light bulb necklace.

Most of the associations I make are quirky, which makes them easier for me to remember, but you may prefer more logical or obvious ones. If so, perhaps you saw a bright light bulb over the movie star's head, indicating she had just thought up a great new idea for a movie.

humans could clearly see a tiger lunging in their direction, they could dodge the predator and have a better chance of surviving. Being visually adept gave some early humans heightened predatory skills, allowing them to better feed themselves and their offspring, which further increased their chances of survival. And their offspring probably inherited that survival advantage by sharing their parent's visually superior DNA.

Many people use visual techniques to teach — one PowerPoint image in a classroom can save a teacher a thousand words. Whether it's a boardroom, classroom, or advertising pitch meeting, visual aids help make a message memorable. However, visual images require a framework in order for us to recall the information later.

Some people are more verbal than visual. Others, like musicians, tend to use their ears more effectively than their eyes. Regardless of your neural predilections, I recommend that you attempt to strengthen your visual skills to fine-tune your ability to create a framework for your memories. (Try Practice Linking Unrelated Words on page 37.)

Name That Face

Learning to recall names is a great place to start training your memory; nearly everyone has difficulty remembering names and faces by the time they reach their 40s and 50s. I took the opportunity to associate names to faces when I memorized 12 new acquaintances at my publisher meeting. You can build this skill too. I recommend starting with just first or last names, and only a few names at a time.

When I meet someone, I usually repeat that person's name back to him or her at the beginning of the conversation:

"Hi, I'm Bill."

"Nice to meet you, *Bill.*"

If possible, I try to mention how the person reminds me of someone else I know with the same name — a very good association tool. If I'm introduced to someone with a foreign or unfamiliar name, I sometimes ask them to spell their name for me. I then try to visualize it spelled out, which helps fix it into my memory. I also try to repeat the person's name again during the conversation, which helps secure it into my memory banks.

It's also helpful to identify a facial feature that stands out and is easy to remember. It could be a warm smile, large nose, or unusual hairdo. It could also be a personality trait or other physical attribute that impresses you. Usually your very first impression sticks the best.

To come up with an image for the person's name, keep in mind that all names can be sorted into two categories: those that evoke an obvious visual image, and those that don't. Last names like Woods, House, Taylor, Hill, Brown, and Hall readily bring an image to mind. Mr. *House* is opening the door to his *house*. Mrs. *Woods* is lost in the *woods*. Ms. *Hall* is walking down a long *hall*.

If a name does not evoke an obvious image, then we need to be more creative and find a visual image that sounds like the name or perhaps even break down the syllables of the name to create two or more visual components. To learn and remember the name of *Today* show weatherman Al Roker, you might visualize him sitting on an *alligator* playing *poker*. You could remember Jimmy Fallon by imagining him at the *gym*, *falling* over a barbell.

Linking a new acquaintance to someone familiar or famous is another good way to frame their name and face. You meet an Elisabeth who has piercing blue eyes that remind you of *Elizabeth Taylor*. (Ms. Taylor actually had violet eyes, but who's doing the remembering anyway?)

You can combine your strategies or stick to one or two. The words and images you think up don't have to be perfect. Sometimes just the mental process of conjuring up images and connecting them is all you need to remember a name for good.

Your Keys Are on the Washing Machine

My friend Jerry owns a busy audio-video business with several offices, and he carries around numerous keys on a large key ring. He doesn't like putting his keys in his pocket because they cause a big bulge. Unfortunately, whenever he's ready to leave the house, he has to search all over to find where he plopped down his keys. Jerry finally decided to follow my advice and choose a *memory place* for his keys. He decided to put them on the washing machine every evening. Now when he leaves for work, he goes right to his keys because he uses the laundry room door to get to his car.

Memory places are tremendously helpful to avoid searching for commonly misplaced objects like glasses, cell phones, wallets, and keys. If you practice putting things in the same place several days in a row, it will become a memory habit and you won't have to think about it anymore. I try to always place my wallet with my keys in a particular drawer in the bedroom so I know where they are, and I get the added bonus of never leaving with one and not the other. Some items may have more than one place. For example, my wife, Gigi, keeps her cell phone either in her purse or plugged into the charger on her dresser. She often puts her purse right next to the charging phone to ensure she won't forget to toss it in later.

Distraction is the most common cause of forgetting things. A busy writer I know told me that she searched her house for 20 minutes to find her misplaced glasses. She finally passed a mirror and noticed that she was wearing them on her head the whole time.

If you do misplace an object, try systematically rerunning your most recent activities in your mind. Then retrace your steps, focusing your attention on each place you might have put the item. Could your broken earring be in the pocket of your jacket that you hung in the closet? Check it out. Perhaps you put it in your purse when it broke at work. If this doesn't work and you're stumped, relax for a few minutes and then retrace your steps again — you may have left something out.

Seeing into the Future: Prospective Memory

Some of the most annoying and common memory slips are forgetting an appointment, leaving an important item at home, or fearing that a missing item is lost or stolen. One of my patients told me a story of how she was driving and talking hands-free to her husband at work. At a red light, she looked over at her open purse and noticed that her cell phone wasn't in it. She panicked — had she left it at home? Did she lose it? She asked her husband to call her right back so she could locate her phone. Of course, when he called, they both realized their mistake. The phone had been in her lap all along.

Most people think that memory functions only to help us recall past events, what neuropsychologists call retrospective memory. But the ability to remember current and future plans, or prospective memory, is also an essential mental skill for taking care of tasks, errands, and everyday business.

Not so many years ago, we relied on pocket organizers or desk calendars to jot down our appointments; today most of us schedule things on our computers and smartphones. However, we don't always enter every single detail about each appointment. Say you have a business meeting and need to bring a relevant file with you. You might get distracted while getting ready, forget the file, and only realize it when you're already there. If this happens more than twice, your prospective memory may need some tweaking.

An effective way to bolster prospective memory is to spend a few moments every morning reviewing your calendar for the day. This memory habit will be reinforced if you pick the same time and place to do it every day, such as before you get out of bed or while you're drinking your coffee. As you review your day, consider the details of each appointment and activity. This

Memorizing Your To-Do List

Have you ever gotten to the market and realized you forgot your grocery list? No problem if you used FOCUS and FRAME to remember your list of groceries or errands. This method builds on your ability to recall unrelated words, since a list of items or errands is merely a list of unrelated words.

Simply think up a story that links together all the words. For example, I was too busy last Saturday to write down a list of the following errands:

Bakery — buy a pie
Dry cleaner — pick up jacket
Watchmaker — change battery in watch
Pet store — buy dog food

To remember these four errands, I created the following story:

While I was taking my dog to the pet store, I got hungry and stopped at a bakery for a pie. My dog leaped for the pie and smushed it on my jacket, which now had to go to the dry cleaner. I checked my watch to make sure I had time, but it had stopped; so I went to the watchmaker to change the battery.

I suggest trying this proven memory method with just a few items at first, but soon you will increase your ability to recall even long lists of unrelated items. Notice that my story was unusual and had lots of action — elements that help make it more memorable.

will help ensure that you are prepared and that you remember to bring everything you need. After just a few days of practice, this new memory habit will become second nature.

It's on the Tip of My Tongue

Not long ago a friend was describing a book she had just read, but she couldn't remember the title. She definitely knew it; it was on the tip of her tongue, but the more she tried to bring it to mind, the more frustrated she got. And this frustration only made it harder for her to concentrate and find the missing word. Of course, the title popped back into her head an hour later, when she was no longer trying to recall it.

Most of us experience these common "tip-of-the-tongue" moments from time to time, and it can be exasperating. The good news is that there are proven techniques that help diminish and even erase these memory slips.

Dr. Timothy Salthouse and colleagues at the University of Virginia in Charlottesville studied 718 adults between the ages of 18 and 99 who were enrolled in the Virginia Cognitive Aging Project. They tested for tip-of-the-tongue errors involving general information by showing photographs to volunteers and asking them to name the famous people, places, and events in the pictures. As expected, tip-of-the-tongue experiences were more frequent in older volunteers than in younger ones, but they *were not* predictive of future cognitive declines. The investigators also measured the volunteers' *episodic memory*, or the ability to recall events in one's own life. Episodic memory also worsened with age, but this type of memory loss was found to be associated with future cognitive decline.

As we get older we acquire more and more information, which increases the likelihood that we'll experience some tip-of-the-tongue memory lapses, and the scientists adjusted for age differences in their statistical analysis of their findings. It's frustrating to forget a name or word that you're sure you know but just can't seem to retrieve. It usually happens because you haven't used the word in the recent past. Relax. The brain cells storing that memory haven't died; they have simply gone dormant and need to be dusted off.

Knowing that these experiences are normal and common annoyances associated with aging helps lower the anxiety that every tip-of-the-tongue moment is an omen of future cognitive decline. People who get nervous every time they can't think of a word only make it harder on themselves to remember it.

By following my system, you can easily lower the frequency of your tip-of-the-tongue moments.

- When a name is on the tip of your tongue and won't roll off, don't push too hard to find it. Simply jot down any details you associate with the name.

- When it's convenient, use your notes to look up the name online or in a book, or ask a friend who may know it.

- Now use FOCUS and FRAME to visually link the name you forgot to one or more of the associations you wrote down.

Here's an example of how it works. The other day my wife, Gigi, and I were talking about old movies, and I mentioned that great satire from the seventies with Faye Dunaway. It was about a TV programming executive who would do anything to get better ratings. I remembered people shouting, "I'm mad as hell and I'm not going to take it anymore," but I couldn't recall the name of the movie. We used my associations to look it up online and groaned when we saw the title *Network*. I then used FOCUS and FRAME to make Network memorable for me: I envisioned Faye Dunaway wearing a hair *net, working* at her desk. I doubt I will ever blank on that title again.

Becoming a Memory Pro

Most people who have become proficient in my methods are more than satisfied to have improved their memory and begun staving off brain aging. But some people are more ambitious and wish to emulate the professional memory wizards who compete in international championships.

Many of these memory masters use a method that takes FOCUS and FRAME to another level: the *Roman Room* method.

Practice Your "Tip-of-the-Tongue" Memory Skills

I did a crossword puzzle today and couldn't remember the name of the author of *Winnie-the-Pooh*. I used my smartphone to look it up on the Internet: of course, A. A. Milne was the author of that favorite children's book. Use FOCUS and FRAME to link the book title to the author's name. Your images might include characters from *Winnie-the-Pooh*. (My images at end of chapter.)

Ancient Roman orators are said to have used this strategy to help them remember what they wanted to say during their speeches. The method links unrelated words or ideas to a familiar series of visual images, such as rooms in a house or objects within a familiar room. You can use this method to remember any kind of list, and it can be very helpful for public speaking.

To try this approach, begin by visualizing some familiar rooms in your house and imagine yourself walking through those rooms on a fixed path. I might start by visualizing myself in my *bedroom*. From there I see myself walking down the *hallway* into the *living room*. I then pass through the *dining room* and enter the *kitchen*. Once I've established my path, I take my mental stroll again, but this time I place an imaginary object representing an idea I want to remember in each room. Lastly, I take yet another mental stroll through my house, reviewing the ideas I wish to recall as I see my imaginary objects in each room.

Here's how I recently used this method to remember the sequence of points I wanted to make in a lecture on Alzheimer's disease. I wanted to start with statistics on the prevalence of Alzheimer's disease, so I envisioned a calculator on my bedroom pillow to help recall numbers or *statistics*. I then walked into the hallway and bumped into a doctor wearing a white coat and stethoscope, reminding me to discuss the *medical assessment* of Alzheimer's. In the living room, I envisioned a large PET scanner that prompted me on my next topic, *diagnostic imaging*. As I passed through the dining room I saw a giant pill bottle on the table — I wanted to discuss *drug treatment* of dementia next. Finally, in the kitchen I saw an athlete jogging in place while eating a big bowl of blueberries, which reminded me to end with a review of *exercise, diet, and other lifestyle strategies* that can delay the onset of Alzheimer's symptoms.

Easy-to-Remember Passwords that Won't Get Hacked

With a multitude of websites and devices to manage, we all need an easy and efficient system to remember our passwords. Without such a system, we may choose only one or two easy-to-remember passwords that might not be so secure.

Here is a method to create passwords that are both safe and easy to recall:

Think up a sentence that has personal meaning to you; for example: My dog is brown. Use the first letters for each word in the sentence as the main body of your password: MDIB. Then, make every other letter a capital letter — this will protect your password by including both upper and lowercase letters: **Mdlb.**

Add a lucky number or symbol in a pattern that is easy for you to remember: **7Mdlb7**. For emphasis, you can bookend the password with exclamation points or other punctuation marks as in: **!7Mdlb7!**

To a would-be hacker it will be tough to crack, but to you it will be memorable.

The *Peg* method is another memory strategy that can help you remember phone numbers and other numerical information. Although we store a lot of this kind of information in our electronic devices, a few numbers are convenient to memorize, like your daughter's cell phone or your driver's license number.

With the Peg method, we associate numbers to visual images that are easier to remember. Start by assigning (and memorizing) a visual image that represents each of the 10 digits.

HERE IS AN EXAMPLE OF A *PEG* SYSTEM I LIKE TO USE:

1 — NECKTIE (looks like a 1)

2 — EYES (come in pairs of 2)

3 — BLIND MICE (there are 3 of them)

4 — TIRES (4 on a car)

5 — NICKEL (5 cents)

6 — BEER (comes in 6-packs)

7 — DICE (lucky 7)

8 — EIGHT BALL (the 8 ball in billiards)

9 — CAT (has 9 lives)

0 — FULL MOON (looks like a rounded 0)

After memorizing these pegs (or your own list), you will be able to create a story to remember any sequence of numbers you wish to memorize. Here's how I would make up a story to represent the following driver's license number:

A2345678

There's a big red *apple* (A) on the desk, and I can't take my *eyes* (2) off it. Suddenly *three blind mice* (3) screech up, burning rubber on their *tires* (4). They ask for a *nickel* (5) to buy some *beer* (6). While drinking, they *roll dice* (7) and the winner gets to hit the *eight ball* (8) into the side pocket.

The story is silly, but once I visualize it a couple of times, I'm bound to remember it.

Your Memory Is Better Already

You've now learned some basic tools to jump-start your memory skills. Early in chapter 1, you tried to memorize a list of unrelated words by creating a story that visually linked each of the words. Now that you've learned FOCUS and FRAME, see how quickly you can memorize the following new list of unrelated words:

Shark
Magazine
Professor
Palm Tree
Row Boat
Airplane
Desk

Is your professor rowing the boat, sitting at the desk, or flying the airplane? Perhaps you see a shark chasing the professor, or maybe the shark is resting against a palm tree surrounded by magazines? The exercise will become easier as you practice, and you will find that your memory skills continue to grow.

More Tip-of-the-Tongue Practice

You're listening to the oldies station and you hear the familiar beat of that rock hit from the late '70s, "My Sharona." You had that album and you know the name of the band, but you just can't think of it. When you find out the band was the Knack, use FOCUS and FRAME so you'll never make this tip-of-the-tongue error again. (My answer at end of chapter.)

These kinds of techniques are very powerful. They not only improve memory right away but they have long-lasting benefits. Our UCLA research group has demonstrated that training in these methods leads to significant improvements in memory performance within weeks. Long-term studies have confirmed enhanced memory and other cognitive gains five years after training. Dr. George Rebok and his colleagues from Johns Hopkins University recently reported significant daily functioning and reasoning benefits in a longitudinal study of 2,832 older adults *10 years* after they took cognitive training classes.

You now know the basics to begin strengthening your memory. As you build your skills in the 2-Week Younger Brain Program, you will find that these methods become second nature and you'll start using them every day.

Mastering Everyday Memory

- Practice the two basic memory tools:

  ‣ FOCUS: Pay attention to what you want to remember.

  ‣ FRAME: Give the information personal meaning to make it memorable.

- Leverage your brain's built-in ability to remember what you see: create visual images for what you want to remember and link them together for better recall later.

- Create memory places to avoid misplacing everyday items like keys and glasses.

- Use visual stories that link together your to-do list items, making them more memorable.

- Conquer the tip-of-the-tongue phenomenon by jotting down a few notes, looking up the forgotten word, and then using FOCUS and FRAME to help remember it next time.

- Try the Roman Room and Peg methods to remember speeches, lists, and frequently used numbers.

 MY ANSWERS TO TIP-OF-THE-TONGUE PRACTICE
Page 44: Practice Your "Tip-of-the-Tongue" Memory Skills
To link *Winnie-the-Pooh* and author A. A. Milne, I see an image of Pooh Bear walking a (for A. A.) mile (for Milne) around a track.

Page 48: More Tip-of-the-Tongue Practice
Whenever I hear the mesmerizing beat of "My Sharona," I imagine myself drumming my *knuckles* to the rhythm of *The Knack*.

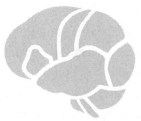

CHAPTER THREE

Cut Stress To Sharpen Your Mind

"There cannot be a stressful crisis next week. My schedule is already full."

—*Henry Kissinger*

IMAGINE YOURSELF RELAXING ON a beautiful beach. The sun is about to set and you can feel a cool breeze on your face. You have no worries, no deadlines. You could drift off to sleep, but you want to stay in the moment and appreciate the brilliant orange, red, and yellow sky as the sun disappears behind the horizon.

Chances are you haven't had one of those truly relaxing moments for a while. Most of us have to schedule vacations to enjoy such experiences, and simply getting to a holiday destination — making reservations, packing, traveling to and from the airport — presents its own form of stress. And, once we've made it to our retreat, we may be distracted from the beautiful vistas by our phones, laptops, or persistent worries that we'd hoped to leave behind.

Stress is a part of everyday life. Sometimes it results from forces outside our control like pollution, noise, accidents, or traffic jams. Other times we bring on our own stress by assuming more responsibilities than we can handle, failing to plan ahead, or getting involved in destructive relationships.

We usually know when we are under acute stress — there's an onslaught of physical and mental symptoms that may include rapid heart rate, perspiration, fear, panic, and worry. Ongoing or chronic stress is more insidious and harder to recognize. Many people believe that if they are not experiencing obvious symptoms, then they cannot be under any real stress. Such unrecognized chronic stress, however, can have profound effects on the body and the brain, contributing to headaches, insomnia, and mood changes, as well as increasing the risk for various illnesses that accelerate brain aging.

Although stress is usually considered the brain's enemy, it isn't always bad. A little bit of stress can motivate us, and learning to cope with setbacks makes it easier to face future challenges. Some intensely stressful experiences can also be thrilling, like racing down a black-diamond ski slope or skydiving at 15,000 feet.

This Is Your Brain on Stress

During my medical studies, I was drawn to psychiatry because of my fascination with the extraordinary power that our minds hold over our bodies. This mental power is particularly dramatic when we look at our physical responses to stress, which are hardwired in our brains and date back to our ancient ancestors' survival strategies.

When these ancestors felt threatened, perhaps by a saber-toothed tiger or aggressive mammoth, the acute stress of that threat evoked a physical fight-or-flight response, releasing cortisol and other stress hormones to their bodies and brains. These hormones caused their hearts to pump faster and transport more nutrients to their neurons, allowing for heightened attention and quick thinking. They had to instantly decide whether to stand and fight or make a run for it.

In our modern world, threats from real predators are rare. Much of the stress we suffer from today is chronic and results from daily aggravations like traffic, work, finances, and challenging relationships. Although our hardwired responses to acute stress remain the same, we no longer require them on a daily basis for survival. Scientific evidence suggests that chronic elevations of stress hormones damage brain cells, impair memory, increase the risk for Alzheimer's disease, and shorten life expectancy.

Just as it has since the days of our early ancestors, acute stress still causes our brain activity to shift from our executive control and thinking centers in the frontal lobe (behind the forehead) to our emotional and reactive centers in the amygdala (beneath the temples). This shift allows us to respond quickly and instinctively to perceived threats — like scrambling to find a missing wallet or avoiding a swerving SUV on the highway — and not getting distracted by any complex problem solving. During this stress-induced, brain-activity shift, it's probably not a good idea to make important decisions because of the frontal lobe's decreased ability to reason through complicated details.

Researchers have injected cortisol into human volunteers and observed significant declines in learning and memory abilities, but when cortisol levels return to normal, their cognitive skills return. In some instances, acute stress has been shown to enhance memory. After intense emotional stimulation, positive or negative, we often remember greater details of events. For example, many of us still recall what we were doing on our wedding day or when we learned about the 9/11 World Trade Center attacks, but not very much of what occurred the previous week. Both animal and human studies point to heightened cortisol levels as the cause of this emotional memory boost.

Some of the psychological symptoms of stress are easy to recognize, such as anxiety, fear, tension, and panic. But stress contributes to other psychological manifestations that are not so obvious, including anger, confusion, depression, impatience, irritability, and memory loss. Stress also leads to physical

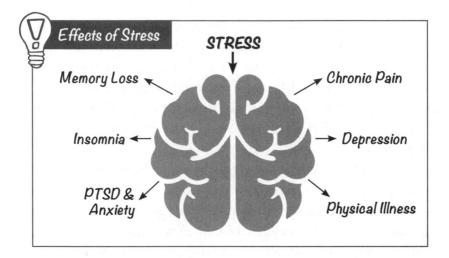

symptoms like pain, appetite change, fatigue, headache, and insomnia. People who suffer from excess stress are more likely to develop heart disease, high blood pressure, and diabetes. Elevated blood pressure can lead to small strokes in the brain, which can impair memory, and people with diabetes have a two-fold greater likelihood of developing Alzheimer's disease.

HOW STRESSED OUT ARE YOU?

If you wish to improve your stress-management skills, it helps to first assess how much stress you are currently experiencing. Place a checkmark in any of the following boxes if the statement applies to you:

☐ I tend to worry about small details.

☐ I usually see the cup half empty.

☐ I often feel tense.

☐ I have trouble concentrating when I am under stress.

☐ I am generally an impatient person.

☐ I usually doubt that things can get much better.

☐ I frequently have trouble sleeping through the night.

☐ Sometimes I have nervous twitches, bite my nails, or pace.

☐ I tend to have a poor appetite.

☐ I often experience headaches, backaches, an upset stomach, or excessive perspiration.

☐ I am usually indecisive.

☐ People notice when I'm tense or anxious.

☐ Sometimes I experience a rapid heart rate or shortness of breath.

☐ I am easily irritated by others.

Add up the number of statements you checked off. If your total is four or less, then you are probably not under very much stress. A score of five to eight suggests moderate stress levels, and a total of nine or more indicates that you may be experiencing an unhealthy amount of stress. The good news is that the higher your score on this brief self-assessment, the greater your opportunity to improve your brain health and memory performance by learning and using effective stress-management strategies.

Stress Affects Memory

Ken and Shirley, both in their late 60s, had finally decided to downsize like so many of their friends had done, and sold the family house in the suburbs. Ken was retiring in a few weeks, and they were looking forward to traveling, spending more time with the grandkids, and fixing up their new condo in the city.

Shirley was busy packing up the house, donating furniture and other things, and sorting through what seemed like tons of memorabilia — kids' artwork, photographs, holiday cards, old datebooks, and more so-called treasures that they wouldn't have room to store at the condo. Her daughters tried to help but it was difficult because Shirley insisted on supervising everything. She wanted to decide what to save, what to get rid of, and how to pack.

Not only was Shirley dismantling their home of 40 years, she had to oversee the improvements on the new condo and learn to navigate a new neighborhood that she had never lived in. Which

---

💡 Hone Your Stress Detector

The next time you are people watching, focus on someone and take note of any body language, gestures, or facial expressions that convey whether or not that person is under stress. Do you notice a wrinkled brow? Is the woman at the next table tapping her foot or restlessly looking around? Does that businessman walking by seem to be late for an appointment? Is he constantly checking his watch? The more you practice, the easier it will become to distinguish between those who seem calm and those who seem stressed out.

Once you're confident in identifying these cues, turn your attention to yourself. Are you sending off stressed-out signals? Are your muscles tense? Are you twirling your hair or pacing without realizing it? If so, take some deep breaths and consider what might be gnawing at you.

---

local market had the best produce? Were there good restaurants close by? Where would she even get her nails done? Shirley's head was spinning. Ken helped out as much as possible, but he was still working full-time and couldn't be around that much.

Shirley also had to deal with her mother who had advanced Alzheimer's disease. She couldn't decide whether to keep Mom at the care facility near the old house or move her to the city so she could be close by. There were so many decisions to make that Shirley started to feel overwhelmed.

Her worries were compounded by the fact that she was having trouble remembering what appointments she'd set up for the day and even where she put her keys half the time. The more forgetful Shirley became, the more stressed out she got. She was scared that she was getting Alzheimer's disease like her mother, and she talked with Ken about it incessantly. He finally told her that if she was really so concerned, she should go talk to a doctor.

When Shirley first came to see me, she was distraught. She told me about her mother and her concern that she had inherited an Alzheimer's gene. She was sure she was having the first signs — missed appointments, misplaced keys, even repeating herself during conversations. When she told me about all that was going on in her life, I said I was impressed that she could remember anything considering how much she had to deal with at the same time.

I gave Shirley a few basic memory tests — word lists, number series — and didn't find any memory issues that were abnormal for her age. We talked about the amount of stress she was under and how stress could sometimes lead to temporary memory loss. This memory impairment, however, could turn into a long-term problem if she didn't do something to cope better with her stress. At the end of the session, Shirley agreed to come back weekly for a while so we could focus on stress-reduction techniques that might help her through the current upheaval in her life.

Within a few more sessions, Shirley learned to recognize when her anxiety was coming on and how to use relaxation techniques to help alleviate it. She began doing deep-breathing exercises, taking short walks one or two times a day, and, most importantly, reaching out for help — like letting her daughters help her with the sorting and packing. Shirley stopped agonizing over every single decision and became more confident in her choices. She wouldn't move Mom for now — any changes could be made later, after things settled down. Shirley rented a small storage space for keeping things she couldn't fit into the condo and didn't want to part with. Becoming decisive and taking action really lowered her anxiety levels.

Soon Shirley reported having an easier time remembering things — she felt sharper and more in control. By the time she stopped seeing me regularly, she had carved out time to take a yoga class twice a week and felt calmer than she had in years.

When people get stressed out, they often become distracted and don't focus their attention on learning new information. Those distractions also make it more difficult to retrieve past memories. Chronic stress can have even more profound effects, not just on memory but on the risk for developing dementia.

Shirley was worried that her memory problems meant she was on the road to developing Alzheimer's disease. She had seen the same symptoms in her mother when Mom's memory started to decline. However, in Shirley's case, it was the stress of the move that worsened her otherwise normal age-related memory slips.

Dr. Lena Johansson and her colleagues at the University of Gothenburg in Sweden studied the brain effects of stress in more than 1,000 women for 35 years. The investigators measured levels of tension, anxiety, fear, irritation, and insomnia and reported that research subjects with greater signs of stress during middle age had higher risks for Alzheimer's disease later in life. They also found that midlife stress predicted more extensive late-life brain abnormalities, including atrophy and scarring of brain blood vessels.

These same researchers also found that the number and duration of midlife stressors were independently linked to late-life dementia risk. So a woman who went through a divorce, lost a job, and had a brother with chronic depression would be more likely to develop dementia than a woman who went through a divorce but kept her job and had no family history of mental illness.

Other studies have shown that individuals who are prone to stress are three times as likely to develop Alzheimer's disease compared to those who are better able to cope. These findings suggest that, despite the varying degree of stress that people face, it is possible to protect brain health from long-term damage through effective stress management.

Even acute stress suffered during childhood, such as experiencing an early parental death, will increase risk for dementia later in life. It may be that these early traumas give rise to long-standing distress that alters the body's stress hormone regulation and eventually damages brain cells. Studies of Holocaust survivors indicate that their stress hormone levels remain elevated even several decades after their traumatic experiences.

A Quick And Easy Stress-Buster

Meditation, yoga, and other stress-reduction exercises help shift our minds away from stress-related, brain-damaging neural activity to more mindful, relaxed, and brain-protective states. Take a couple minutes to try this exercise for a quick mindfulness boost:

- Sit in a comfortable chair, place your feet flat on the floor, and allow them to point slightly outward.
- Rest your hands on your thighs with your palms facing up and close your eyes.
- Take some deep, slow breaths in through your nose, exhaling through your mouth.
- Feel your body relax as your mind grows peaceful.
- Continue inhaling and exhaling for another minute or two, then open your eyes.

One or more episodes of severe trauma can lead to more persistent forms of anxiety, such as post-traumatic stress disorder (PTSD). Patients with this condition often experience recurring flashbacks and nightmares. Some studies suggest that stress hormone responses in these patients may be overactive, making the brain hyperresponsive to any fearful stimuli. In addition to the intrusive, unwanted memories of the traumatic events, PTSD patients frequently complain about difficulty remembering everyday events that are not emotionally charged.

Investigators at the University of California in San Francisco found that patients with PTSD scored lower on cognitive functioning tests. The scientists noted that risk factors under the patients' control were contributing to their lower scores, suggesting that increased exercise, better diet, more education, and other healthy lifestyle strategies could improve their stress-related cognitive symptoms.

Neural activity in the brain's frontal lobe appears to account for the flashbacks and nightmares in PTSD. The brain's hippocampus (temporal lobe) puts memories into context and is involved in the emotional memories of PTSD. Suppression of hippocampal activity may contribute to PTSD symptoms.

Tackle Mood Problems

Sometimes chronic stress can lead to depressions that are more persistent than the transient lows people may feel from day to day. At some point in life, about one in every five of us will experience a depression that interferes with daily activities, but these depressions can improve with psychotherapy, antidepressant treatment, or both.

A complicated mix of chemical imbalances in the brain contributes to depression. This is significant because our brain chemistry is sensitive to psychological and social triggers. The neurotransmitter serotonin does not function as well or becomes depleted in depression, which is why antidepressants that boost serotonin improve symptoms.

Even if someone has a genetic predisposition to depression, psychological stress clearly plays a role. Psychodynamic therapy can alleviate symptoms of depression. It helps put the patient's

---

Recognizing Major Depression

To determine if you or someone you know is suffering from a depression that may respond to treatment, look for four or more of the following symptoms:

- Feelings of sadness or hopelessness
- Difficulty sleeping through the night or too much sleep
- Loss of interest in usual activities
- Feelings of guilt
- Fatigue and low energy levels
- Poor concentration and memory complaints
- Reduced or increased appetite or weight
- Thoughts of suicide

Someone may suffer from only two or three of these symptoms and still need help if the symptoms are severe enough. Also, an older person may be depressed and experience symptoms that don't look like a typical depression. That person may not feel sad at all but instead be overly concerned about his physical ailments and memory loss. In such cases, weight loss, insomnia, and other physical symptoms of depression can help pin down the diagnosis.

psychological conflicts into perspective and increases their understanding of how past experiences influence present behavior. Cognitive behavioral therapy is another effective talk therapy that improves mood by challenging depressed patients' negative thinking patterns and helping them to change unwanted behaviors.

The structure and function of your brain may contribute to your risk for depression. Brain scan studies of depressed patients have demonstrated reduced volumes in regions that control emotional regulation, including the amygdala, hippocampus, and some areas in the frontal lobe, which manages empathy and impulse control. The more doctors understand the physiology of depression, the better they can target specific treatments. Dr. Helen Mayberg and colleagues at Emory University found that depressed patients respond best to cognitive psychotherapy when low activity levels are observed in the anterior insula (a region that regulates our emotional reactions). Patients with higher insula activity have better outcomes with antidepressant medication.

If depression is left untreated, it often worsens memory abilities. Research also points to depression as a risk factor for developing future dementia and Alzheimer's disease. Patients with mild cognitive impairment (MCI) who are also depressed are twice as likely to develop dementia as MCI patients who are not depressed. Some older patients who are both depressed and cognitively impaired may initially improve with antidepressant medication, but eventually their cognitive impairment worsens and stops responding to the medicine.

Sometimes people get depressed when they realize their memory skills are declining, but our UCLA studies suggest that symptoms of depression may actually be a physiological response to neurodegeneration already going on in the brain. Dr. Anand Kumar and I performed brain PET scans on older patients with major depression and found elevated levels of amyloid plaques and tau tangles — the same abnormal protein deposits observed in the brains of Alzheimer's patients.

High Anxiety

For some people, stress causes anxiety, not depression. Worry, fear, and panic distract people from focusing their attention and remembering effectively. Full-blown anxiety disorders, such as panic attacks, PTSD, and agoraphobia can be crippling.

High anxiety increases stress hormone levels in the brain, which can contribute to stroke risk. Dr. Maya Lambiase and associates at the University of Pittsburgh followed more than 6,000 volunteers for over two decades and noted a 33 percent higher stroke risk for volunteers who reported greater levels of anxiety. We also know that anxious people are more likely to smoke and have high blood pressure — two more explanations for why anxiety is linked to stroke.

Stress-Pain Cycle

An old friend of mine suffered from back pain on and off for years. His back tended to flare up when something stressful was going on in his life — a breakup with a girlfriend, a sudden drop in the stock market, or some other problem he couldn't fix.

Stress and pain often go hand in hand. When people are emotionally stressed, they tend to notice preexisting pains more. Conversely, chronic intense physical pain makes most people feel stressed, anxious, and depressed.

Emotional stress signals the body's sympathetic nervous system to release adrenaline and cortisol. These stress hormones trigger muscle tension that can cause headaches, back pain, temporal mandibular joint (TMJ) syndromes, and other discomforts. Digestive tract activity slows down, which can trap gas in the abdomen and lead to stomach cramps and indigestion. Chronic stress also shifts the body's inflammatory system into high gear, aggravating any existing physical conditions like heart disease or asthma. All of these physical responses just lead to further emotional distress.

Suffering any type of acute pain is stressful, but that pain serves an important function — it signals the brain that the body is injured and needs attention. However, when pain is allowed to linger and become chronic, it can limit a person's physical activity levels and interfere with learning and memory.

An individual's underlying brain structure can predict whether their pain will be temporary or chronic. Dr. Vania Apkarian and her scientific team at Northwestern University Feinberg School of Medicine used MRI scanning to study the brains of patients experiencing lower back pain. They found that the outer rim of their brains, known as the grey matter, was consistently smaller in patients whose pain persisted for a year. However, effective treatment can reverse both brain shrinkage and chronic pain. Dr. David Seminowicz and associates at the University of Maryland found that an 11-week course of cognitive behavioral therapy improved symptoms in patients with chronic pain, and increased the volume of the grey matter in their brains.

With many forms of stress, simply talking about feelings with supportive friends and family members can improve one's state of mind. However, chronic pain sufferers who constantly dwell on their symptoms tend to distance people and create dysfunctional relationships that leave the patient feeling isolated instead of supported. As a result, many pain sufferers become uncomfortable talking about their symptoms, which can leave them feeling even more isolated.

Treating pain effectively lowers stress, and sometimes antidepressant drugs can reduce symptoms of depression and pain. When you are less depressed, you are less aware of aches and pains in your body, and learning better ways to relax will improve symptoms of pain.

A Good Night's Sleep

Restful sleep is crucial for keeping our brains young, but stress often impairs our ability to sleep through the night. Sleep deprivation not only leads to fatigue, it also impairs concentration, learning, and memory. Insomnia and fretful sleep are associated with higher rates of diabetes, obesity, and heart disease — all conditions that can compromise brain health. Studies show that people deprived of just two hours of sleep will experience short-term

> ## Stress-Reduction Break
>
> Lie down or sit in a comfortable chair. Take a few deep, slow breaths and then close your eyes. Begin to relax each muscle group in your body, starting with your toes and feet. Release any tension you are holding there, and as you continue breathing slowly, let that sense of relaxation move up through your calves and into your thighs. Next, let the relaxation spread through your pelvis and abdomen. Gradually relax the muscles in your chest, arms, and hands. As you next relax your shoulders and neck, you may wish to move them around a bit to release any tension there. Now relax your jaw and facial muscles.
>
> Finally, take another deep breath, exhale, and open your eyes. Your body will feel relaxed and your mind will be tranquil. This is a very effective way to quickly de-stress any time of day.

memory deficits. This is a very common problem since at least 50 percent of adults suffer from some form of insomnia and are unable to get enough sleep.

During sleep, the brain consolidates memories, which improves recall abilities the following day. As daybreak approaches, about 20 percent of our sleep cycle is rapid eye movement, or REM, sleep, which is vital to mental health. During REM sleep, our brains are dreaming, and studies show that a reduction in this important stage of sleeping can cause mental exhaustion.

Sedative medications that are used to treat insomnia suppress REM sleep. When people stop using these medicines, they often experience extremely vivid dreams, a phenomenon known as rebound REM.

Researchers have discovered neural changes that occur when sleep is compromised, and these neural changes can affect mental clarity and brain health. Swedish scientist Christian Benedict and colleagues at Uppsala University found that when volunteers are deprived of a night's sleep, they have temporary elevations in blood levels of molecules typical of brain damage. Dr. Adam Spira and colleagues at Johns Hopkins, Bloomberg School of Public Health reported that poor sleep quality and shorter sleep duration are associated with higher levels of amyloid protein, one of the abnormal brain deposits of Alzheimer's.

When we don't get enough sleep, our brains become inflamed. Tiny inflammatory cells attack normal brain cells, and when chronic, this process can contribute to the neurodegeneration found in Alzheimer's disease. However, after a good night's sleep, this inflammatory process is reversed and inflammation lessens significantly. Snoring and fretful sleep increase the risk for metabolic syndrome, another condition that can lead to cognitive impairment.

When we're awake and doing our usual mental work, our brain cells metabolize, or use up oxygen and nutrients. This process creates metabolites and debris that must be cleared out of the brain because they are toxic to neurons and can contribute to Alzheimer's disease. Sleep is essential for clearing out this metabolic waste. Animal studies at the University of Rochester and New York University confirmed that sleep increased activity of the brain's waste-removal system.

Difficulty sleeping is also a symptom of depression. When depressed patients receive standard treatment — psychotherapy, medication, or both — their sleep patterns improve. A newer strategy for treating depression addresses the sleep issue head-on, by using cognitive behavioral therapy for insomnia. This structured program helps patients pinpoint thoughts and behaviors that compromise their sleep and teaches them to substitute new behaviors that promote restful sleep.

Top 10 Stress-Busting Strategies

It's impossible to erase all of life's stressors, but we can learn strategies to reduce them. My UCLA research team used brain PET scans to show that people who achieve greater psychological well-being display less evidence of the abnormal brain proteins found in Alzheimer's disease. That study suggests that lowering stress levels and achieving mental well-being may protect the brain from Alzheimer's disease.

To help keep your brain young and healthy, try some or all of my top 10 stress-busting strategies:

1. MEDITATION

The sight of someone sitting in a lotus position and chanting "om" was rare in the Western world until the late 1960s when the Beatles met the Maharishi and learned about Transcendental Meditation. Today, this 5,000-year-old practice is popular everywhere.

Meditation not only lowers stress levels and improves mood, it strengthens neural circuits and increases mental focus. A recent MRI brain study indicated that an eight-week program consisting of only two hours of weekly meditation protected the brain's hippocampal memory center from atrophy. It also improved neural connections between different memory areas that are susceptible to Alzheimer's-like neurodegeneration.

Meditation increases awareness and attention by focusing the mind on a sound, image, or movement. In *transcendental meditation*, people concentrate on a single syllable or word, known as a mantra; in *mindfulness meditation*, they focus attention on sensations and breathing.

Some people initially find it difficult to quiet their minds and meditate, but with practice it becomes easier. To get started, set a timer for five minutes and try the following steps:

- Sit cross-legged on the floor or in a comfortable chair.

- Close your eyes and begin to breathe deeply and slowly.

- Focus on your breathing while allowing your body to relax.

- If your mind wanders, simply bring your attention back to your breathing.

- You may choose to concentrate on a mantra instead of your breathing.

As your skills improve, set your timer for longer sessions.

2. YOGA AND TAI CHI

Many Westerners get antsy when they try to meditate and prefer stress-reducing techniques that involve a physical component. The ancient spiritual practice of yoga integrates movements, poses, and breathing routines that provide a relaxation response while boosting flexibility and balance. Yoga not only reduces stress, it improves symptoms of depression, anxiety, and chronic pain. Although yoga poses appear static, they provide aerobic and strength training benefits that bolster brain function. Yoga also protects the brain by lowering levels of inflammation.

Tai chi is a traditional Chinese practice that promotes relaxation and balance. Many tai chi sequences look like martial arts in slow motion, and they avoid the jarring motions of other types of exercise that can aggravate joint problems. Recent research suggests that tai chi boosts immune function and reduces symptoms of fatigue, pain, anxiety, and depression.

3. EXERCISE

The endorphin boosts and anti-inflammatory effects of cardiovascular conditioning can quickly reduce stress levels and cause an immediate improvement in mood. Creating an exercise routine — a daily visit to the gym before work or perhaps a brisk walk after dinner — is an effective stress-management strategy. Also, a spontaneous mini-workout like climbing a few flights of stairs or marching in place for a few minutes may be just the trick to break up a particularly stressful day. The physiological effects of exercise can reduce chronic pain. Workouts that strengthen targeted muscle groups and increase flexibility may further reduce pain by helping to avoid injuries.

4. CUTTING BACK ON MULTITASKING

Our brains crave stimulation, and we are drawn to new technologies that provide novelty and entertainment. With so many new gadgets and electronics in our lives, many of us are tempted to multitask. We may respond to a text while in a meeting, or talk hands-free on the phone while driving. Our multitasking skills can be honed with practice, but too much multitasking causes stress. Although multitasking gives us the perception of greater mental efficiency, in truth our brains cannot attend to several tasks at the same time. When we multitask, we are actually rapidly switching our focus from one single task to another. Scientists have found that rapidly switching mental focus increases the time it takes to complete each task and results in a higher rate of errors.

Technology expert Linda Stone first described a related problem, *continuous partial attention*, wherein people constantly monitor multiple devices with only partial attention, waiting for the next blast of exciting stimuli. Both multitasking and partial continuous attention can contribute to mental fatigue, distraction, and memory impairment. Over time, these stressful mental states increase cortisol levels, which can worsen memory and mood.

Becoming mindful about multitasking is the first step to controlling it. Setting aside regular off-line periods and turning off your devices are helpful strategies for limiting its impact. Also, scheduling certain times each day to answer e-mails may eliminate the compulsion to constantly check your in-box.

5. LIGHTEN YOUR LOAD AND LAUGH

Many of us are people pleasers — we have trouble saying no to others. But making too many commitments can put us under a lot of unnecessary stress. It's easy to agree to do something that seems minor, but little tasks add up and together they can cause stress and anxiety about all the details that need attending to and the time it will take to do so.

To lighten your load, make a list of the tasks and errands you plan to complete tomorrow. Review your list and try to pick one or two items you can skip, delegate, or postpone. This process can provide immediate relief and may open up your schedule for additional stress-reduction exercises.

Having a good laugh offers immediate tension release and helps us feel closer to each other. Hearing a funny joke can quickly improve our mood and may even offer new insights and perspectives on a troubling situation.

Laughter's benefits result in part from increased endorphin release and improved blood flow to various memory centers in the brain. Just watching a rerun of a favorite sitcom can be enough to snap us out of feeling stressed or down. Research indicates that even forcing ourselves to laugh can lighten our mood. Dr. Charles Schaefer at Fairleigh Dickinson University found that when he directed volunteers to smile or laugh for up to a minute, they experienced substantial mood boosts.

6. RESTFUL SLEEP

We know that a good night's sleep optimizes brain health, but as we get older, we don't require as much sleep: a 20-year-old may need at least eight hours each night, while a 70-year-old may need only six hours. Regardless of your age, if you are experiencing insomnia or fretful sleep, try some of the following sleep strategies:

- **Avoid daytime naps.** These may be invigorating but can lead to less tiredness at bedtime. To break the afternoon nap habit, try walking or exercising during that time to better sleep at night.

- **Limit evening liquids and caffeine.** Drinking liquids in the evening may cause you to awaken in the night if your bladder calls. If you are sensitive to caffeine, avoid coffee, tea, cola sodas, or even chocolate, which can keep you awake due to their caffeine content.

Talking to Yourself Reduces Stress

Almost all of us talk to ourselves from time to time. Sometimes we do it when we're happy; other times when we're tense. Talking out loud to ourselves has been shown to lower stress levels and calm us down. Recent studies indicate that if you address yourself by name in the third person, your self-talk is even more effective in reducing anxiety and building confidence.

Here are a few examples of helpful self-chats for various situations:

- **Speaking in public:** "Remember to make eye contact, Gary, and speak clearly."
- **Applying for a job:** "They'd be lucky to hire someone like Shirley. Shirley has the talent and the ability."
- **Competing in sports:** "Focus on your forehand, Susan. It's your best tennis stroke."
- **Proposing marriage:** "You know she loves you, Steve. She will definitely say yes."

- **Create a restful environment.** Make sure your bedding, pillows, and sheets are as comfortable as possible. Keep the bedroom quiet, dark, and cool.

- **Take it easy in the evening.** Some people have trouble settling down after watching an exciting movie or sports event, so try to avoid too much mental stimulation before bedtime.

- **Use relaxation methods.** Deep breathing, imagery, meditation, or anything that relaxes you can help you drift off to sleep. Once you're in bed, keep your body in a comfortable and still position.

- **Train your brain to sleep.** The following technique has worked for several of my patients: Get into bed at the same time every night, and don't eat or watch television while in bed. Take a few moments to get comfortable and relax. If you have not fallen asleep after 20 minutes, get up, leave the bedroom, and either read a book, listen to music, or watch television. Once you begin feeling tired, go back to bed and try to sleep again. If you're still not asleep in 20 minutes, get up and leave the bedroom again. Return to bed when sleepy and attempt to fall asleep for another 20 minutes. You may need to continue this method throughout the night, but make sure you don't nap the next day. After sticking to this strategy for a day or two, many people are able to train their brains to sleep through the night.

7. GET ORGANIZED

Stress often results from poor organization and planning. Disorganization and clutter can increase stress hormone levels and impair memory and brain health. However, research shows that even hoarders with extreme clutter issues can improve with treatment. Getting organized and reducing clutter leads to greater productivity and a better sense of control in our lives. It also makes it easier to find things.

Clutter generally builds up over time even when we try to avoid it, so creating regular decluttering habits is helpful. Set small, attainable goals — instead of attempting to declutter the entire house, start out with a drawer or other area that you use often. Donate or throw away things you no longer need. Rarely used items should be stored in places you don't have to access daily. Try planning one day each week when you can spend a little time decluttering a different area. This will likely reduce your stress and give you a sense of accomplishment.

Creating daily planning habits reduces stress. Simply reviewing your calendar and to-do list each morning can have a major impact and doesn't take much time.

8. ACUPUNCTURE

This ancient Chinese practice involves the insertion of thin needles into the skin at specific pressure points throughout the body and is used to treat a variety of physical and mental conditions. The traditional explanation for acupuncture's effectiveness is based on the theory that the needles unblock chi — energy flowing through the body along pathways known as meridians, which allows the body to heal. Western experts believe that the needles stimulate areas with high concentrations of nerve endings, which elevates endorphin levels in the brain, thereby reducing pain and lowering stress.

Acupuncture is an effective treatment for a variety of pain syndromes and stress-related conditions, including depression and anxiety. Some practitioners enhance the needles' effects with mild electrical currents or heat. People who are shy of needles might consider acupressure, a form of touch therapy that stimulates the same body points as acupuncture, but substitutes finger pressure for needles.

A recent functional MRI study looked at the effects of acupuncture on brain activity in patients with Alzheimer's disease. It showed that acupuncture increased brain activity in regions controlling memory and cognition, suggesting its potential positive impact on these mental capacities.

9. POSITIVE ATTITUDE AND RELATIONSHIPS

Learning to be more upbeat can improve our brain function. Optimists report less stress, fewer physical and emotional difficulties, and higher energy levels than pessimists. Positive thinkers also avoid depression, which can compromise brain health if not adequately treated.

Scientists have identified regions in the brain's frontal and temporal lobes that control many optimistic feelings. Functional MRI studies have demonstrated the changes that occur in these brain areas when an optimistic person observes a scary face or perceives a threatening situation. These studies suggest that people with a positive attitude actually have brain wiring that helps them cope well with adversity.

Cognitive training can help pessimists become more optimistic by teaching them positive responses to events that trigger negative emotions. Making an effort to be more extroverted, learning to forgive, and avoiding negative thinking by focusing on one's strengths helps people maintain a positive attitude. Social psychologist Amy Cuddy and colleagues have shown that correct posture and assertive body language can boost self-confidence.

People with a positive outlook are more likely to attract and spend time with other optimistic people. Maintaining meaningful relationships with supportive friends and family members lowers stress hormone levels, helps reduce anxiety, and decreases the risk of dementia. Talking about our worries helps put them into better perspective; just having a stimulating 10-minute conversation with a friend can boost cognitive abilities.

10. ASKING FOR HELP

Many people have trouble asking for help, often because they fear that others may refuse or let them down. Researchers found that anticipated rejection can increase brain inflammation, which may compromise memory if it becomes chronic. Despite such hesitation, reaching out for help has been hardwired in

---

Lower Stress To Protect Your Brain

- Try meditation to reduce stress and lift your mood.
- Get regular physical exercise to boost brain circulation and endorphin levels.
- Limit multitasking to improve efficiency, diminish distractions, and bolster memory performance.
- Experiment with proven stress-busting activities like yoga and tai chi.
- Try laughing to gain perspective on everyday worries.
- Learn strategies for getting a good night's sleep.
- Get organized and reduce clutter for a greater sense of control.
- Try acupuncture to help reduce pain and stress.
- Keep a positive attitude and strong social relationships.
- Learn to ask for help.

our brains through evolution — it offered our early ancestors a survival advantage. Scientists have identified the brain networks involved in asking for help: the amygdala's emotional control center and the frontal lobe's planning region.

If your stress levels are affecting your daily life, talk with your doctor. Medication, psychotherapy, or a combination of both have been effective for many conditions and can dramatically improve symptoms and overall well-being.

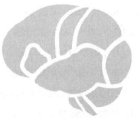

CHAPTER FOUR

Get Smart with Brain Games

"My brain? That's my second favorite organ."
—*Woody Allen*

BARRY POPPED THE FINAL two pieces of his jigsaw puzzle into place to complete the picture of four horses running through a field. He called out to his wife, Ruthie, that he'd finished another one.

She yelled back from the kitchen, "Congratulations, honey. Now you can work on that brain-training program I signed us up for."

Barry's feelings of accomplishment vanished — he always got frustrated when Ruthie pushed her interests on him. They had both retired the previous year and resolved to keep doing things that challenged their minds — their doctor said it would help stave off memory loss and other effects of brain aging. Barry liked that they were traveling more and taking ballroom dancing lessons, but those brain games on the computer weren't his thing. He knew they were supposed to stimulate his mind, but they weren't fun and made him feel stupid. Barry preferred to stick with his jigsaw and Sudoku puzzles.

The next Sunday, their son Alex came over for dinner. During dessert, Ruthie mentioned the brain games program, and Alex was intrigued. He worked for a video game design company and knew a lot about computers. Barry tensed up just hearing them talk about it, and Ruthie sensed his discomfort.

"Dad won't even give the games a fair try."

"I did try them," Barry responded. "I just don't like them."

Alex took his coffee over to the computer. "Dad, sign in for me so I can check this thing out."

Barry grumbled something under his breath and typed in his password: *B - A - R - R - Y.*

Alex tried filling in the missing answers to a match game that Barry had begun. "I see what you mean, Dad. It's frustrating when you can't pick out the answers before the clock runs out," Alex said.

Barry gave Ruthie an "I told you so" look.

"Wait a minute. You have the level set on advanced, Dad. You should start out on beginner and work your way up. No wonder you don't like it," Alex laughed.

Alex changed the level and quickly beat the computer at its own game. Barry sat down next to Alex. He took the mouse and clicked on the word game icon. A partially filled-in Scrabble board appeared, as well as seven letters to use to make a new word.

Barry made the word "brown" and got 12 points. The computer played next, and Barry rapidly responded with a 15-point move. Ruthie started clearing the dishes.

"I'll help you in a minute, honey," Barry said, filling in yet another word on the computer Scrabble board. "I guess this isn't so bad . . ."

Alex smiled and went to help his mother do the dishes.

Barry's problem was that he started playing brain games at a level that was beyond his abilities. It frustrated him so he lost interest. Our brains enjoy a good challenge, but if a task is too challenging, we tend to give up and do something else. Likewise, if a game is too easy, we usually get bored quickly.

Studies of working memory and intelligence showed that not all subjects improve from brain games. When volunteers were asked to play a game that was too demanding, their cognitive scores did not improve. However, when they played a game geared to their particular level of play, their memory and intelligence scores increased.

Most mornings I enjoy doing the newspaper's daily crossword puzzle. I know that the crosswords are easiest on Mondays and grow more challenging as the week progresses. Over the years I've come to realize that I am a Tuesday-through-Thursday puzzler. I usually find Monday too easy and Friday fairly difficult.

To get an idea of how a simple brain game can progress from easy to challenging, below are two versions of a popular game that exercises verbal fluency, or the ability to come up with words.

Beginnner Level

Set a timer for two minutes and then, using the letters below, jot down as many words as you can containing three or more letters. Use each letter only once in each word.

ESMTA

I was able to come up with 17 words in two minutes, but when I spent more time I got 25 words. (See my answers at the end of the chapter.)

Intermediate Level

Now that you've fired up your verbal fluency skills, see if you can take it to the next level. Set your timer for three minutes, but this time use the following seven letters to form as many three or more letter words as possible.

AEIORAM

This exercise works out the areas of your brain that control logic and language. Your frontal lobe allows you to see patterns that make it easier to form words. Perhaps you'll try to come up with as many words as you can starting with the letter "A," then build words with the next letter "E." Try not to keep checking your timer, because your amygdala's emotional center may get charged up and distract you with anxiety.

There are several ways to make this exercise more challenging, such as substituting less frequently used consonants like "X" or "Z," decreasing the amount of time allotted, or changing the number of letters allowed in each word.

Mental Workouts for Brain Fitness

For many years we've known that physical exercise keeps our bodies strong, and now scientific evidence suggests that mental exercise keeps our brains young. In fact, any brain-stimulating activity that tweaks your neural circuits — painting, reading, traveling, doing puzzles, learning languages, searching online, and more — can enhance your cognitive abilities.

Studies have shown that people who graduate college have a lower risk for developing Alzheimer's disease than those who never got a degree. Some experts believe this is due to certain people inheriting "smart genes" that preprogram them toward a college trajectory, and that their neurons simply fare better with aging. But we don't need a college degree to help keep our brains young with stimulating activities.

Research indicates that we can all build more brain muscle with mental exercise. Scientists looked at laboratory animals raised in stimulating environments — cages with mazes, toys, and other stuff that mice find mentally exciting. Compared to mice raised in standard-issue cages, the mentally stimulated animals demonstrate better cognitive abilities — they are able to find the cheese at the end of a maze faster than the control mice. Their brain's hippocampal memory centers were found to be substantially bulkier, and a bigger brain is a healthier one.

These kinds of discoveries have spawned a whole new category in the fitness industry: brain training. Instead of breaking a sweat on the treadmill or pumping iron at the health club, people of all ages are now training their neural circuits at the local brain gym or doing their mental aerobics at home using brain games, puzzles, computer programs, or websites in order to fight off brain freezes and senior moments. The recent interest in brain fitness has paralleled the rapid growth of electronic media devices that allow us to play almost any game or puzzle we can find on a disc or online.

Too Much Technology

Our fascination with these gadgets can have repercussions. Distractions due to multitasking, as well as the stress caused by paying continuous partial attention to our devices, can hamper brain function and memory abilities (see chapter 3). Although new technologies offer more opportunities to exercise our brains, many people overuse their devices. Our UCLA research team has been studying the effects of technology on the brain, in part because of the link between screen time and behavior issues in children and teenagers. Watching too much television or spending too much time playing video games is associated with attention deficits, symptoms of attention deficit hyperactivity disorder (ADHD), and poor academic achievement. We're still not sure if the screen time causes the problem — some experts contend that kids who have worse cases of ADHD just happen to like watching more TV. But even if screen time doesn't cause ADHD symptoms, it appears to worsen them.

When my son was a teenager, I remember growing concerned that his video game playing might not be good for his brain development. One Saturday afternoon, I heard him playing some fantasy-action video game for nearly two hours straight. The game's silly noises and music were getting to me, and I finally yelled to him, "Harry, that's enough with the video games. Come downstairs right now and watch TV with me!"

By the time I finished that sentence, I realized how ridiculous I sounded, but I assumed that watching a public television program with his dad would be better for his developing brain than playing the same old video game over and over again. What I didn't realize was that Harry was playing the game online with his friends and having ongoing conversations with them — the social interaction alone was probably providing a brain benefit.

Although some of my concerns were valid, not all brain games are created equal. We're now learning that some online and computer games can actually improve memory, increase problem-solving skills, and even make us smarter.

Brain Games That Boost IQ

Recent studies indicate that certain games can train a form of short-term memory that is crucial for problem solving and a component of what we define as intelligence quotient, or IQ. Neuropsychologists measure IQ using one of several standardized tests, including the Stanford-Binet test or the Wechsler Adult Intelligence Scale (WAIS). People with an IQ score of 100 are considered average — about 95 percent of the population score between 70 and 130 on these standardized tests.

Initial studies of twins found that identical twins were more likely to have similar IQs than fraternal ones. These results led many experts to assume that IQ was largely an inherited genetic trait and a relatively stable aspect of mental function. The prevailing thinking was that most people were born with average, above average, or below average intelligence and their IQ remained relatively constant throughout life. This assumption that IQ is fixed has been challenged by a series of studies indicating that basic memory exercises can bolster IQ scores.

Although an individual's IQ is inherited to some extent, the environment and experiences throughout life, especially early in life, influence IQ scores. For example, breastfeeding and musical training during childhood are associated with higher IQ scores.

Intelligence can be defined as comprising a range of mental functions including attention, reasoning, visual and spatial skills, and verbal skills — all cognitive abilities that can be assessed with pencil and paper tests. Higher scores on IQ tests are associated with greater academic and professional achievement. However, emotional intelligence, or our ability to understand how feelings impact our thinking, also guides our actions and can be just as important to success in life as IQ.

IQ measures cognitive intelligence, which has two major components: crystallized and fluid. Knowledge we acquire from learning is defined as *crystallized intelligence*. It improves with

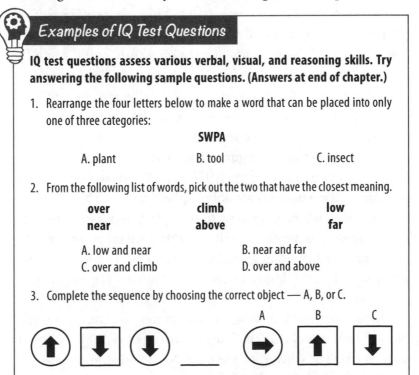

Examples of IQ Test Questions

IQ test questions assess various verbal, visual, and reasoning skills. Try answering the following sample questions. (Answers at end of chapter.)

1. Rearrange the four letters below to make a word that can be placed into only one of three categories:

     SWPA

     A. plant   B. tool   C. insect

2. From the following list of words, pick out the two that have the closest meaning.

     over   **climb**   **low**
     near   **above**   **far**

     A. low and near   B. near and far
     C. over and climb   D. over and above

3. Complete the sequence by choosing the correct object — A, B, or C.

age because we continually learn new information over the years. *Fluid intelligence*, by contrast, allows us to solve problems and understand abstract ideas.

Drs. Susanne Jaeggi, Torkel Klingberg, and other investigators studied the impact of brain training on memory and intelligence. They found that playing specific computer games could improve both attention and working memory, which led to better fluid intelligence. Working memory is short-term memory that allows us to temporarily organize and manipulate new information. This is the kind of memory we use to hold information briefly in mind to call a phone number we've just heard or solve a simple math problem.

Dr. Jaeggi's group found that when elementary school students played a brain-training video game that improved their working memory and attention abilities, their fluid intelligence scores showed significant improvements. The video game was based on principles used in the well-known, card-matching game of concentration, and the students only needed to play the game for about 20 minutes, five days a week to raise their IQ scores.

By training working memory, fluid intelligence benefited as well. This makes sense since solving problems requires us to use our working memory to hold various bits of information in mind long enough to figure things out. This useful skill also helps us navigate life's many challenges. When we organize and use information well, we are able to plan for things like appointments and what we may need to bring to those appointments. Other studies indicate that the working memory and intelligence boost from brain games is not unique to children — college students, middle-aged people, and seniors appear to enjoy the same benefits.

These memory-boosting match games are based on the N-back test, a tool that challenges someone's recall for a sound or image recently heard or seen. An N-back test might ask you to recall the location of a sound or color presented just before

Concentration Card Games With N-Back Boost

Deal four cards face up and focus your attention on remembering one card in particular. Turn the cards over, distract yourself for 20 seconds, and then turn over the card you wanted to remember to ensure it's in the correct position. Build your concentration abilities gradually by trying to remember the position of two cards, then three, and so on until you master the basic four-card memory task. Next increase it to six cards, then eight.

Once you've strengthened your attention and working memory skills with this first game, try a classic game of concentration: Remove four matching pairs (e.g., two aces, two sevens, etc.) from the deck. Shuffle the eight cards and lay them out face down in two rows. Turn over two cards and see if you were lucky enough to get a match. If you did, take those cards out of play. If not, try to remember the placement of those cards and turn them face down again. Turn over a different card and see if it matches one of your previous cards. If it does, remove the matched cards from play — if you can remember the location of the first card. If not, turn over another new card and hope you get lucky. Again, if you've gotten a pair, take it out of play and repeat. After completing this match game with 8 cards, move on to 10, 12, and more, as you gradually build your memory skills. Before you know it, your working memory and problem-solving abilities will be sharper than ever.

the most recent (1-back), the time previous to that (2-back), or the time just before that (3-back), and so forth.

To build even bigger brain muscle, you can try a dual N-back task, which asks you to remember both a sound and an image presented simultaneously. You can get a sense of what these games are like by visiting www.brainworkshop.sourceforge.net or www.soakyourhead.com. You can also find a free smartphone app with a version of a dual N-back game by searching the key words "IQ boost" online. If you are trying to cut back on your computer time, you may be able to improve your working memory and IQ off-line with a simple deck of cards.

Shake Up Your Brain Training

In right-handed people, the brain's left side, or left hemisphere, usually controls language and reasoning skills. Word games help build this left hemisphere, while mazes and jigsaw puzzles can bolster the right hemisphere that controls visual skills and orientation.

The brain loves variety, so cross-training, or challenging your brain with different types of exercises will make your mental aerobics more interesting. Simply brushing your teeth with your nondominant hand is fun because it changes things up. Our minds are always curious about things that are new or different. TV reruns and yesterday's headlines are dull, but new information grabs our attention and brings pleasure to our neurons. Even when something is not completely new, it only needs to be a little different from what we saw or did before for our brains to enjoy it.

Neuroscientists think that our attraction to novelty and variety is hardwired in our brains. Unfamiliar stimuli and new mental challenges activate a brain region known as the *reticular formation*, located in the back of the brain where it connects with the spinal cord. This novelty-seeking region may have developed and evolved because rapidly attending to unfamiliar sights and sounds improved our ancient ancestors' ability to detect predators — there was an adaptive advantage to being able to quickly spot an attacker.

As I developed the brain-training exercises for the 2-Week Younger Brain Program, I took into account the fact that our brains prefer variety to repetition. Rather than asking you to do multiple repetitions of the same brain exercise, I want you to shake things up by cross-training your brain just as you may cross-train your body when working out. Many physical fitness trainers agree that it's best to cross-train your body, or incorporate different forms of exercise into your routine. For example, combining aerobics and weight training promotes better overall fitness than just one approach alone.

When doing brain exercises, it's a good idea to alternate right brain training with left brain training. Depending on the particular brain game you play or mental skill you activate, it is possible to energize two or more entirely different brain regions that are responsible for a particular function.

When I do my morning newspaper puzzles, I like to switch them up so that I exercise different brain regions. I may begin with a number puzzle like Sudoku or KenKen, and then shift to a word puzzle like a crossword or word jumble. This strategy makes my mornings more interesting and fun.

Try the following two puzzles and notice how it feels when you switch mental tasks that activate different brain regions. Start with a Sudoku puzzle, which will activate your left brain math skills as well as your right brain visual-spatial skills. In case you've never played Sudoku, note that the goal is to complete a 9 x 9 grid that is subdivided into nine, 3 x 3 boxes. Some squares

Try Sudoku

	2	7	3	8		5		6
4		5			6	8		1
1		8	4				3	7
3	7	2	1	4		6		
		4		9				2
6		9	5		7	4	8	
8	4		7	6		2		9
2				9			4
	9	6	2	1				8

Word Jumble

Quickly unscramble the following sets of letters to make eight words. Then draw lines between the words that go together. Your lines should create a number that may remind you of lunchtime. (Answer at end of chapter.)

lepap   *kfro*   *krecor*   *tinsec*

nlsuite   *tiruf*   *ihrca*   *yluebtrflt*

will already have numbers in them. Try to fill in the rest of the squares so that every row, column, and 3 x 3 box contains the numbers 1 to 9 only once. The difficulty level of the puzzle depends on how many of the digits are already placed in the grid when you start, and where they are placed. The fewer numbers already placed, the harder the puzzle. Try this beginner-level Sudoku. (Answer at end of chapter.)

If you're new to Sudoku, it may take a little while to get the hang of it, but with practice you will likely come up with strategies for solving these puzzles. You might start by focusing on the 1–9 digits within the rows, the columns, or the 3 x 3 grids. You can even lightly pencil in possible answers. When you no longer need to pencil in answers, your working memory will help you hold various number options in mind for brief periods. As you build your skills, you can increase the difficulty level to keep your brain engaged.

Now switch gears and pump up your neurons with the next word jumble game. It will tweak your frontal lobe language center, as well as other regions in your cortex that help sort information into categories.

When Neurons Talk, Minds Strengthen

Focused mental workouts can stimulate specific brain regions, but most mental activities require the interaction of several brain areas at once, and this brain cross-talk strengthens an

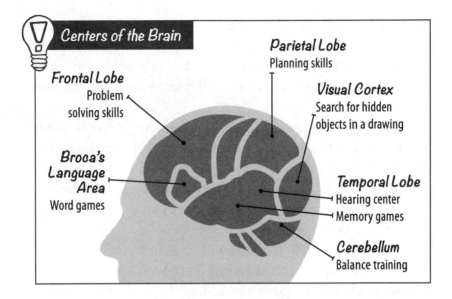

Centers of the Brain

Frontal Lobe
Problem solving skills

Broca's Language Area
Word games

Parietal Lobe
Planning skills

Visual Cortex
Search for hidden objects in a drawing

Temporal Lobe
Hearing center
Memory games

Cerebellum
Balance training

array of neurons. In our UCLA research studies, we often ask volunteers to learn and remember word lists. That mental task specifically targets the frontal lobe language region and the hippocampal memory center in the temporal lobe, but other brain areas get involved as well. Various types of sensory input activate different brain areas: when you *read* a word, your visual cortex in the back of your brain fires signals to the language area in your frontal cortex; if you *hear* the word, your auditory temporal cortex will feed messages to your frontal cortex (see figure above).

When messages are transmitted across brain networks, it exercises our neurons and neural circuits become stronger and larger. The region that extends through the center of the brain and separates the right and left hemispheres is known as the corpus callosum. A plump and healthy corpus callosum means that the right and left brain are communicating effectively.

In most right-handed people, the right brain is the visual and emotional hemisphere and the left is more analytical and verbal. The opposite is true for left-handers. If the corpus callosum is working properly, our analytical and verbal left brain abilities, such as reasoning, speaking, writing, and reading, remain in sync with our right brain functions, such as reading maps, enjoying music, recognizing faces, and perceiving depth, humor, and emotions.

Studies of the corpus callosum indicate that bigger is better when it comes to intelligence: the more bulk it has, the higher your intellectual capacity. Albert Einstein's brain had a particularly hefty corpus callosum connecting his right and left brain regions, allowing him heightened ability to imagine and manipulate spatial information.

Other research indicates that with repeated practice, we can boost several mental functions and observe corresponding increases in the brain regions controlling those functions. Scientists have found that London taxi drivers with 20 years of driving experience have significantly larger right hippocampi compared with novice cabbies. The old-time drivers' right brain map-reading skills and hippocampal memory centers have become bigger and more proficient after decades of driving.

Although these enhanced skills and brain bulk are specific to a practiced task, they transfer to other related tasks as well. We'd expect those experienced British cabbies to also excel at solving maze puzzles — a visual-spatial challenge that also requires short-term memory skills. Some mental activities, such as learning to play a musical instrument, stimulate multiple brain regions that provide cognitive advantages. Experienced musicians who have played their instruments longer demonstrate better academic performance. Extensive musical training has been shown to increase the volume of gray matter in brain regions that control motor and hearing abilities.

If music is not for you, you might consider studying a foreign language to encourage your brain cells to communicate and bulk up. Learning a new language increases the size of the hippocampus, and studies show that bilingual people have a lower risk for developing Alzheimer's disease than those who speak only one language. Conversing in two or more languages exercises brain circuits, especially when translating words from one tongue to another.

Searching Online Builds Brain Muscle

Many people now spend more time online than watching television, and those hours of searching the Internet can build neural muscle. Just searching online for the address of a new restaurant will activate your neural circuits.

Our research team has studied what occurs in the brain when someone searches online. We looked at brain activity in people who were naïve to the experience of searching online to see what happens to their brains after they gain some familiarity with it. We recruited a dozen older adults who had never searched online and matched them by age and education to a group that was Internet savvy. Using a functional MRI scanner, we measured both groups' brain activation while performing a simulated Internet search. We then compared those patterns to the volunteers' brain activation while reading a book.

People who had prior Internet search experience showed significantly greater neural activity when searching online compared with those who had never searched online before. Reading a book, however, caused relatively minimal activity in both groups. We also found substantial changes in brain activity after the Internet-naïve subjects gained experience searching online. After practicing only an hour each day for a week, the Internet-naïve volunteers demonstrated significant increases in neural activation in their frontal lobes while searching online. The increases were noted in brain regions that control decision making and short-term memory.

When people search the Internet, they instinctively adjust their search pace according to their personal style for absorbing

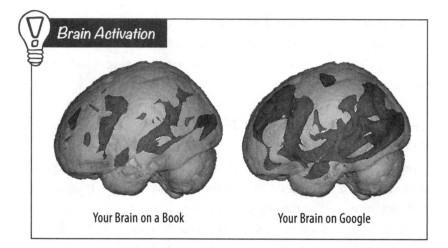

Brain Activation

Your Brain on a Book   Your Brain on Google

new information. Some people like to rapidly scan sites, quickly moving forward or backward while searching. Others prefer a more leisurely pace to explore specific information in greater depth on one web page at a time. No matter the search style, as someone practices and becomes more efficient at searching the Internet, we'd expect to see less neural activity. That may be why studies show lower neural activity while volunteers read a book. Reading is a mental task that most people know very well. Their brains' proficient reading skills use up less mental energy than searching online (see figure above — darker areas indicate where the brain is working during the task).

Training Multitasking Skills

Since the link between mental stimulation and lower dementia risk was established, numerous brain-game websites have popped up online, and although a lot of these games are fun to play, not all of them do too much to improve your general cognitive abilities. Of course, if you play any game long enough, your score will get better, but you still may forget your password to the site, or even where you put your tablet or laptop. If your goal is to improve your mental efficiency, it's important to find games that actually provide benefits.

Some online brain games have been tested systematically, and a few have demonstrated effectiveness in improving specific cognitive abilities. My UCLA colleagues recently found that older adults who played the computerized Dakim BrainFitness game a half hour each day enjoyed improved memory skills after several months of consistent play. And the longer they played the game, the better their memory scores got.

Keep in mind that computers, smartphones, and other gadgets tend to distract our focus and tempt us to multitask. And although attending to multiple tasks at the same time can make us feel more efficient, studies show that repeatedly shifting our attention between tasks actually takes up more time and leads to increased errors.

Despite the distractions and inefficiencies of multitasking, recent research showed that there are certain types of video games that can help strengthen our multitasking skills so we make fewer errors. Dr. Adam Gazzaley and his colleagues at the University of California, San Francisco, asked volunteers to play a video game that involved driving a simulated car on a winding road with distracting street signs. While attempting to keep the car in the correct lane, players had to identify certain street signs that popped up and ignore other irrelevant signs. The scientists used brain scans to test the volunteers' multitasking skills before and after training on the game and found that older adults between ages 64 and 80 could train their brains to multitask and focus attention at the same level as 20-year-olds who had not been trained.

Games People Play

Many popular games that people already enjoy playing actually train specific mental skills that enhance everyday task performance. For example, playing a language-skill game like Scrabble improves executive functioning as you plan your word-placement strategy, and playing a visual-spatial game that challenges

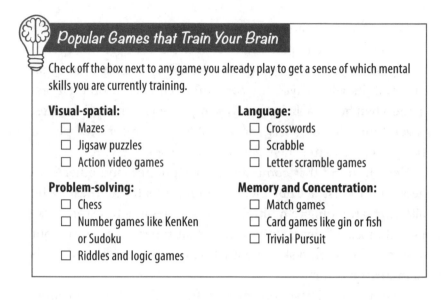

Popular Games that Train Your Brain

Check off the box next to any game you already play to get a sense of which mental skills you are currently training.

Visual-spatial:
- ☐ Mazes
- ☐ Jigsaw puzzles
- ☐ Action video games

Language:
- ☐ Crosswords
- ☐ Scrabble
- ☐ Letter scramble games

Problem-solving:
- ☐ Chess
- ☐ Number games like KenKen or Sudoku
- ☐ Riddles and logic games

Memory and Concentration:
- ☐ Match games
- ☐ Card games like gin or fish
- ☐ Trivial Pursuit

you to fit several items into a tight space teaches great packing skills for traveling. To help keep our brains young, we should strive to play a variety of games that target different mental skills.

Brain Games: Getting Started

The 2-Week Younger Brain Program introduces brain games and exercises that will activate your neural circuits and bolster your mental acuity skills. As you gradually build your skills, you'll find that these games get easier, so you can progressively increase the challenge level. The following are some sample brain games that boost a range of cognitive functions to help keep your mind limber and sharp. (For additional game websites, see appendix 1.)

Beginnner Exercises

Warming up: Any familiar task requiring the use of your dominant hand (right hand if you are right-handed) can become a challenge if you switch to using your nondominant hand. Right-handers, try printing your name with your left hand. After printing both your first and last name, try writing it in cursive.

1. **Right brain exercise: Counting Squares** — Count up the number of squares in the figure below. Hint: Be sure to count the squares within the squares.

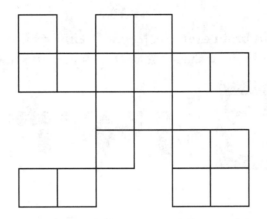

2. **Left brain exercise: Changing Words** — Begin with the word WALL and change one letter at a time until you get to the word FIRM. Each change must be a proper word.

W A L L

— — — —

— — — —

— — — —

F I R M

3. **Right brain exercise: Numbering Toothpicks** — Arrange the three toothpicks below into the number nine (without breaking or bending them).

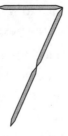

4. **Left brain exercise: Letter Scramble #1** — Try to come up with as many words as you can from the following letters. Use each letter only once in each word.

I R N A B

5. **Right brain exercise: Jigsaw Brain Break** — Keep your right brain in shape today. Which piece fits in the puzzle:

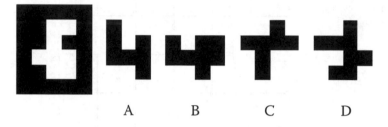

A   B   C   D

6. **Whole-brain exercise: Sorting Words** — The brain naturally organizes information into categories to make memory more efficient. It's easier to remember two fruits and two vegetables than four individual items. Strengthen your sorting skills by identifying the three categories of the nine items below:

CHICKEN	**PLIERS**	**MAGAZINE**
WRENCH	**NOVEL**	**YOGURT**
BIOGRAPHY	**SALMON**	**VICE**

 Intermediate Exercises

Now that you've had a chance to warm up your neural circuits, let's step up the challenge to the next level.

1. **Right brain exercise: Visual Connecting** — Here's another brain workout to enhance your right brain visual-spatial skills and your frontal lobe's ability to split your attention between two mental tasks. In the figure below, draw a continuous line that connects the number 1 to the letter A, then A to 2, then 2 to B, then B to 3 and

so on, until you can no longer continue the numerical or the alphabetical sequence. If you get this right, give yourself a star.

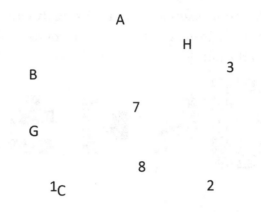

2. **Left brain exercise: Finding Colors** — Rearrange the letters to find the four colors mixed up below. Hint: Only one is a primary color.

   RAIGET   ENOLYL   OVGOEN   LEWRE

3. **Right brain exercise: Straight Line Drawing** — See if you can draw four straight, connected lines that pass through all of the eight dots below. Each line must touch each dot only once, and you should not lift your pencil from the paper while drawing the lines. Hint: free yourself up from one of the usual assumptions you use to connect the dots.

4. **Left brain exercise: Letter Scramble #2** — Write down as many words as you can with three or more letters,

using the letters below. Each letter can only be used once in each word.

I M R O A E

5. **Right brain exercise: Jigsaw Brain Break #2** — Your right brain needs a little more of a workout. Which piece fits in the puzzle?

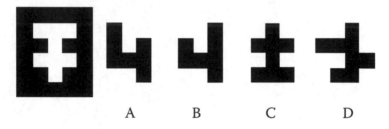

A   B   C   D

6. **Left brain exercise: Proverb** — All the vowels have been removed from the following proverb, and the remaining letters have been clustered into groups of three or four letters each. Replace the vowels and reveal the proverb.

TWH   DSRB   TTRT   HNN

Advanced Exercises

You're now warmed up enough to start using your entire brain (both the right and left hemisphere) to try to solve these brainteasers.

1. **Letter Scramble #3:** — Try to come up with as many words as you can (two or more letters) from the following letters:

O G E U N R Y

Extra Credit — A seven-letter word from this letter scramble and a five-letter word from **Letter Scramble #1** will remind you of a book you are reading.

2. **Hypothetical Country** — A large nation has an overpopulation problem. For socioeconomic reasons, families prefer

to have boys over girls, and most families continue to have children until the birth of a son. If we assume the same probability for girls and boys to be born, what will be the ratio of girls to boys in this country after 10 generations?

3. **Visual Connecting #2** — In the figure below, draw a continuous line connecting the first odd number 1 to the first letter of the alphabet A, then to 3 (the next odd number) and to the next letter of the alphabet B, then 5 to C, and so on until you can no longer continue the sequences. If you succeed, you will have drawn a recognizable structure.

4. **Sequence Recognition** — See if you can recognize the incomplete sequence below and add four lines to complete it.

5. **Odd One Out** — Keep your sorting skills in top form. Pick out the word below that does not belong in the category suggested by all the other words. You will need to unscramble each word first to identify the main category.

ANTK   PJEE   XITA   UNBMARIES   BREOBM

6. **Finicky Frank** — Frank has very eccentric tastes. He is a big fan of football, but hates rugby. He very much likes beer, but despises ale. He drives a Ferrari, but wouldn't be caught dead in a Lamborghini. Based on Frank's finicky tastes, would he prefer skiing or cycling?

7. **Sequence Recognition #2** — Here's another sequence that includes verbal skills, visual skills, and reasoning abilities involving pattern recognition. Figure out which tile completes the sequence.

ILK	HERE	GAP
FINE	ELF	DINE
CON	BAIL	

APT	ALPS	COIL
A	B	C

DIN	NAIL	IRK
D	E	F

Optimizing Your Brain Game Experience

• Brain exercises should be challenging and fun to keep you playing for the long haul.

  ‣ If a game is too hard, dial it back to an easier level.

  ‣ If a game becomes too easy, increase to the next level of difficulty or switch to another game.

• Search the Internet to exercise your neural circuits.

• Your brain likes variety, so vary your mental workouts to bolster both sides of your brain and diverse regions.

• Try games that enhance specific mental abilities, including multitasking and fluid intelligence.

ANSWERS TO SAMPLE GAMES AND PUZZLES

Page 77: Beginner Level

EAT, EAST, EATS

SAME, SATE, SEAM, SEAT

MAS, MAT, MATE, MAST, MASTE, MATES, MET, MEAT, MEATS, META, METAS

TAM, TAME, TAMES, TASE, TEA, TEAS

ATE

Page 77: Intermediate Level

AERO, ARE, ARM, AIM, ARE, ARM

ERA

IRE

ORE

RAM, RIM RIME, REAM, ROAM

MAR, MARE, MER, MIRA, MIRE, MORA, MORE, MORAE

Page 81: Examples of IQ Test Questions

1. C (WASP)

2. D

3. B

Page 85: Sudoku

9	2	7	3	8	1	5	4	6
4	3	5	9	7	6	8	2	1
1	6	8	4	5	2	9	3	7
3	7	2	1	4	8	6	9	5
5	8	4	6	9	3	1	7	2
6	1	9	5	2	7	4	8	3
8	4	3	7	6	5	2	1	9
2	5	1	8	3	9	7	6	4
7	9	6	2	1	4	3	5	8

Page 86: Word Jumble

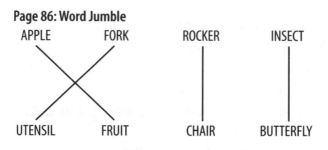

APPLE   FORK   ROCKER   INSECT

UTENSIL   FRUIT   CHAIR   BUTTERFLY

Page 92: Beginner Exercises

1. Counting Squares
   I counted 21 squares.

2. Changing Words
   WALL, WILL, FILL, FILM, FIRM.
   (You may have come up with different words.)

3. Numbering Toothpicks

4. Letter Scramble #1
   I, IN
   RA, RAN, RIB RAIN
   NA, NAN, NAB
   A, AN, AIR
   BA, BAN, BAR, BIN, BARN, BRAN, BRAIN

5. Jigsaw Brain Break
   B

6. Sorting Words
   Tools (pliers, wrench, vice); reading material (magazine,
   novel, biography); edibles (chicken, yogurt, salmon)

Page 94: Intermediate Exercises

1. Visual Connecting

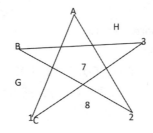

2. Finding Colors

GREEN, ORANGE, VIOLET, YELLOW

3. Straight Line Drawing

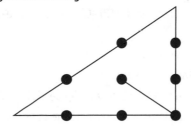

4. Letter Scramble #2

I was able to spell out the following words.
You may find more.
IRE
MAR, MARE, MIRE, MORE
RAM, REAM, RIM, RIME, ROAM
OAR, ORE
ARM, ARMOR
EAR

5. Jigsaw Brain Break #2

C

6. Hidden Proverb

Two heads are better than one.

Page 96: Advanced Exercises

1. Letter Scramble #3

ON, OR, OY, ONE ORE, ORG, ONER

GO, GEN, GUN, GUY, GYN, GONE, GORE, GREY, GONER

EON

UN

NU, NUG

RUE, RUN, RUG, RUNG, ROUGE

YO, YON, YOU, YOUNG, YOUNGER

Extra Credit

The seven-letter word is YOUNGER, and the five-letter word
is BRAIN.

2. Hypothetical Country

The ratio of girls to boys will still be 50:50. The odds of
having a boy or girl will remain the same even if all families
adopted the strategy of no more births after their first son
is born.

3. Visual Connecting #2

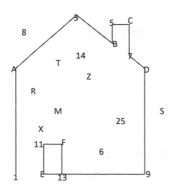

4. Sequence Recognition
Correctly placing four lines gives you the sequence of alphabet
letters from T to Z, upside down.

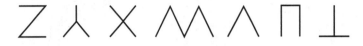

5. Odd One Out
The correct answer is XITA (TAXI), since all the other
unscrambled words are military vehicles (TANK, JEEP,
SUBMARINE, BOMBER).

6. Finicky Frank
Frank would prefer skiing since he only likes words that
contain double letters.

7. Sequence Recognition
Tile A, which contains the word "Apt," completes the
sequence. The first letter of the word in each tile is in reverse
alphabetical order ("I" from "Ilk" is after "H" in "Here," etc.).
The words also alternate from three to four letters.

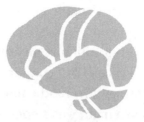

CHAPTER FIVE

Food for Thought

"I come from a family where gravy is considered a beverage."

—*Erma Bombeck*

REMEMBER A LOT ABOUT my family dinners when I was a kid. My father would get home from work around six. I'd feed the dog, and then my sisters and I would wash up and take our usual seats at the table. Every meal began with a salad tossed in Thousand Island dressing — I was never sure where those islands were.

Our entrée depended on what night of the week it was. Monday was fish sticks, Tuesday was hamburgers, Wednesday roasted chicken, Thursday lamb chops, and so forth. I looked forward to Sunday nights because I loved hot dogs and beans.

Mom's side dishes varied from green beans to French fries. If it was fries, there was always a mad dash for them, followed by a heated debate between us kids over who got the most. Ketchup, my favorite condiment, was heaped on everything.

One reason I remember those dinners in such detail is that my mother created a routine, so we knew what to expect each night. We developed nutritional habits — some of them good, others not so much.

I learned more about nutrition as an adult and revised many of my family meal traditions. I still combine proteins and carbohydrates at most meals, but my food choices have changed. Although my mother's fish night was a good idea, fried fish sticks don't do much to promote brain health. Grilled salmon is a much healthier substitute. My family would have fared better if our vegetables had been steamed or grilled rather than sautéed in butter. And French fries? On occasion and in moderation they don't do much damage, but brown rice is a much better alternative.

When I was growing up, people were already aware of the importance of nutrition to physical health. We had Jack LaLanne telling us to avoid processed foods and take vitamins, and we knew that eating right helped keep muscles strong and immunity levels high and protected us from obesity and age-related diseases like hypertension, heart disease, and diabetes. But back then, little was known about how nutrition affects mental acuity. We now know that what's good for the body is also good for the brain, and the idea that "we are what we eat" really rings true when it comes to our cognitive processing.

Changing Our Brain's Eating Habits

Keeping our brains young often involves altering the food habits we picked up as kids. We tend to crave the old, familiar, and comforting foods we grew up with, so adjusting our diets can be challenging at first, but with a little practice it gets easier.

Neuroscientists have studied what happens in our brains when we are engaged in the internal struggle over whether to indulge in a yummy-looking piece of cake or instead resist the temptation and opt for fresh fruit. Scientist Cendri Hutcherson and collaborators at the California Institute of Technology (Caltech) used functional MRI scanning to reveal which neural

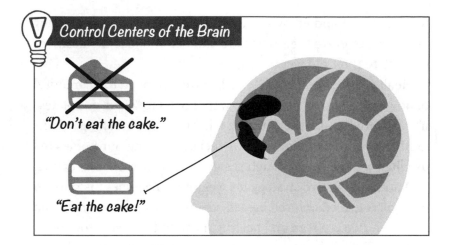

Control Centers of the Brain

"Don't eat the cake."

"Eat the cake!"

circuits encourage self-regulation and which circuits sabotage those efforts.

The scientists found that the decision whether to devour or resist a pleasurable treat is made in our prefrontal cortex — the front part of the brain that regulates most decision making. When we do indulge in the cake, the prefrontal's ventromedial region (in the middle of the forehead just above the eyes) takes charge. But when we are able to resist the fat- and sugar-filled cake, the prefrontal's dorsolateral area (near the temples), which places more value on health than taste, wins the day.

Food Fight in the Brain

When we are stuck in old, unhealthy food habits, it's tough to resist the repeated chants of our ventromedial cortex: "Eat the cake, eat the cake." But with a little awareness and self-discipline, we can break those old habits, and doing so actually adjusts our brain's neural circuitry, making it easier to stick with new healthy choices.

When I help patients form better eating habits to regain and extend their youthful brain function, they often rave about the results once they're gotten beyond their initial resistance. These patients not only experience greater mental clarity, they begin to lose weight and enjoy sounder sleep. In just two weeks, they even start to crave their new food choices and lose the desire to go back to their old ways.

Healthy food choices are vital, but we also need to be mindful of how much we eat. Many of us were raised to "clean our plates" if we wanted dessert, and that is a habit worth breaking. Maintaining awareness of how full we feel and letting our bodies tell us when we have had enough is a good way to avoid overeating.

Another effective strategy for weight management is portion control. A grilled chicken breast, steamed vegetables, and a cup of brown rice is a lean and healthy meal, but if we eat too much carbohydrate-rich rice, we may consume unnecessary calories. Portion control is a real challenge when dining out. A lot of restaurants serve huge portions, and it's hard to resist finishing everything in front of us. Splitting an entrée with someone else is a good way to control those portions, and saying no to the bread basket helps cut calories too.

Food, Mood, and Addiction

What we eat has a big impact on how we feel and think, and, conversely, our thoughts and feelings affect our food decisions. Many of us spend a lot of time planning, preparing, and thinking about our meals. If this mental energy results in well-balanced daily nutrition, it's well worth it. But for some people, thoughts and feelings about food can get out of control, leading to unhealthy eating patterns that can become self-destructive.

I recently got a call from Karen, a middle-aged woman I had treated five years earlier. She told me that she had just gone through a messy divorce and felt like her life was out of control. We made an appointment for her to come in the next day.

I remembered that when I first treated Karen, she was a busy executive in a large marketing firm and was stressed out by the overlapping demands of her job and family. Back then Karen's stress had led to a fairly serious online gambling habit. I had worked with her to control her gambling addiction, stop smoking, and find healthier ways of dealing with stress, such as yoga and meditation. Apparently things were not going so well for her now.

When she entered my office the following day, and I immediately noticed how different she looked — she had gained at least 30 pounds since I saw her last. She sat across from my desk and thanked me for giving her an appointment so quickly. I asked her how I could be of help.

She dropped her eyes. "I know I've put on some weight, Dr. Small, but that's the least of my problems."

"What's going on, Karen?"

"My life is falling apart. I mean, with my husband leaving, the ridiculous pressure at work, and my teenager's demands on my time, I feel totally out of control."

"Have you been gambling?"

"God no, but now I have this eating problem. The more anxious I get, the more I want to eat — especially at night when I'm alone."

Karen's eyes welled up and I pushed the tissue box toward her. I recalled that she used to be quite trim; in fact, she had been somewhat compulsive about her weight and fitness. Clearly she still had compulsive tendencies — her focus had shifted from gambling to overeating.

"I can understand how upset you feel, Karen."

"Of course I'm upset," she said. "Bruce up and divorces me, I'm sick of my job, and I've turned into a big fat slob. Who wouldn't be?"

"What happened with Bruce?"

Karen sighed. "I guess it was coming for a while. He was always complaining that I didn't give him enough attention — all I cared about was work, the kids, and my parents. Can you imagine a grown man getting jealous if I talked to my mother on the phone for 10 minutes?"

"And you couldn't work out your differences?"

"Not after he started dating his legal assistant," she snapped. "But I started gaining weight way before that — not long after I stopped gambling."

When Karen gave up her compulsive gambling, she felt she had overcome her addiction problem. But by refocusing her obsession onto food, she had apparently just replaced one unhealthy addiction with another. I wanted to help Karen recognize and understand this process so she could gain some power over it.

"Do you see any kind of pattern here, Karen?"

"What do you mean?"

"Well, it seems that when you stopped gambling, you switched to a new fixation — food. You replaced one compulsive behavior with another."

She shifted in her seat. "They're not the same at all. I was able to just stop gambling — cold turkey. I can't completely stop eating."

"That's true," I replied. "But I recall you telling me that gambling gave you a sense of control in your life — only you could decide when to play or when to quit."

"So?"

"You also control how much food you eat, and control issues may be a recurring issue for you."

It was my experience that people usually didn't choose to deal with an addiction until they experienced a crisis and were forced to face it. I wanted to help Karen get a handle on her eating problem before she developed a health crisis. She admitted that even though binge eating calmed her nerves and took her mind off her other problems, she always felt horrible and guilty afterward. She wanted help.

Karen had what is called binge-eating disorder, a new classification in the American Psychiatric Association's Diagnostic and Statistical Manual of Mental Disorders (DSM), which recognizes food addiction as a clinical diagnosis, just like drug and alcohol addiction. Just like any addict, when food junkies see their object of desire or get stressed out, it triggers them physically — heart rate slows and brain blood vessels dilate — and the preprogrammed behavioral response kicks in: binge eating.

I began seeing Karen weekly and after a month of treatment she started attending an Overeaters Anonymous 12-step program. She felt uncomfortable there at first but soon found that talking with other recovering food addicts made her feel understood and helped her avoid binging.

As therapy progressed, Karen learned about healthy food choices and portion control. We identified many of the stressors in Karen's life that made her anxious and triggered her to binge-eat, and she began to see how her desire to control every part of her life — work, marriage, family — was an impossible goal to achieve. Soon Karen was able to let go of her food obsession and lose weight, without refocusing on a different unhealthy behavior.

The same neural pathways that reinforce dependence on alcohol or drugs also control compulsive behaviors involving any type of pleasurable activity, including eating, gambling, sex, and shopping. When we feel euphoric, our brains get flooded with dopamine, a chemical neurotransmitter that modulates our brain's reward system.

Addicts compulsively crave, seek, and attempt to re-create the same sense of elation they first felt when they began the addictive behavior. Dopamine stimulates the brain's pleasure centers, causing addicts to want to repeat those actions — over and over again, even when they are no longer experiencing the original pleasure and may be aware of negative consequences. And, as an addiction takes hold, the brain's frontal lobe, responsible for judgment and decision making, loses ground.

Most of us don't suffer from extreme food addictions like Karen, but we all have nutritional habits that affect our eating choices. To maintain brain health, it's important to learn about the right foods to eat and understand how our feelings about food can impact our dietary habits.

Excess Weight Ages the Brain

Although the health dangers of being overweight and obese are widely known, a majority of people continue to live with excess body fat. According to the World Health Organization, more than one billion people worldwide are overweight and 300 million are obese. These individuals have an increased risk for illnesses that can age the brain and accelerate cognitive decline.

More than 50 percent of obese people also have a medical condition called *metabolic syndrome.* Its symptoms include central obesity (excess body fat around the belly), elevated blood sugar, high triglycerides and blood pressure, and low HDL or "good" cholesterol levels. People who suffer from metabolic syndrome are at increased risk for developing heart disease, diabetes, and memory loss.

Central obesity increases inflammation throughout the body, including the brain. When inflammatory brain cells attack normal brain cells, it can cause neurodegeneration and cognitive decline. Studies show that on average, people with central obesity have smaller brains, which heightens their risk for dementia.

Body mass index, or BMI, is a measure of body fat based on a person's height and weight. Healthy weight is defined by a BMI between 18.5 and 25. The BMI for overweight or pre-obese people usually ranges between a 25 and 30. Obesity is often defined as a BMI of 30 or more.

 WHAT'S YOUR BMI?

The following formula will help you calculate your BMI:

(weight in pounds x 703) ÷ (height in inches)²

▶ For example, if you weigh 150 pounds and you are 5 foot 8 inches (i.e., 68 inches), then your BMI is: $(150 \times 703) ÷ (68)^2 =$ 22.8 (which is in the normal range). If you would like to use

your computer to make the calculation for you, visit
www.cdc.gov and search for BMI Calculator.

Scientists at Toulouse University in France found that people with high BMIs had difficulty processing some types of information: their abilities to learn word lists and substitute numbers for symbols were slower compared to people with normal body weight. The investigators also found that people with a higher BMI at baseline displayed greater cognitive decline after five years of follow-up.

People with high BMIs have a harder time controlling their appetite. As BMI rises, the frontal lobe neurons that manage impulse control stop functioning normally, which can lead to trouble resisting unhealthy food temptations. High BMI also increases the risk for insulin resistance. Insulin transports sugar from the blood to the cells, so when cells are insulin resistant, they are less responsive to that insulin and they can't absorb sugar correctly. Insulin resistance can lead to diabetes and increased risk for cardiovascular disease.

It is possible to have a normal BMI and still suffer from obesity because BMI doesn't account for body composition (the proportion of fat to muscle inside the body). In other words, someone with a normal body weight may still have a high and unhealthy fat level inside their body. The term *TOFI* (thin outside, fat inside) has been used to describe this condition, which affects about 12 percent of adults, and can be diagnosed with a body CT or MRI scan. Unless they have had such a scan, these individuals may not be aware of their greater risk for metabolic syndrome and type 2 diabetes. Common symptoms of diabetes include frequent urination, excess thirst and appetite, and unusual weight loss or gain. Anyone concerned about their risk for diabetes should consult their doctor.

Learning that excess body weight ages the brain motivates many people to change their eating habits and boost their

Meal-Planning Brain Game

You mention to your boss that he and his wife should come by your new place for dinner sometime, and he says they are available that very night. You don't have time to go to the market, so you have to use what's already in your refrigerator and pantry. Because your boss is a fitness enthusiast, you want to impress him by making a health-conscious meal. You know you have enough vegetables to prepare a salad and frozen yogurt for dessert, but you have to improvise the entrée. Once home, you find you have the following ingredients below. As quickly as possible, check off the ingredients you'll use to create a main course, and then write the name of that course at the bottom.

____ Ground beef	____ Onions	____ Whole milk
____ Chicken breasts	____ Butter	____ Sugar
____ Hamburger buns	____ Mushrooms	____ Olive oil
____ Bacon	____ Tomatoes	____ Cornflakes
____ Mayonnaise	____ Whipping cream	____ Cheddar cheese
____ Whole-wheat pasta	____ Frozen cheese ravioli	
____ Cream of mushroom soup		

Main course_____

If you used the ground beef, buns, cheddar cheese, and bacon to make bacon cheeseburgers, they probably tasted good, but you didn't impress your boss with your healthy eating. A tasty and nutritious alternative would have been grilled chicken breasts served with whole-wheat spaghetti and fresh tomato sauce with onions and mushrooms in it.

brain health. New research shows that losing weight leads to improved mental function and memory abilities. Dr. John Gunstad and coworkers at Kent State University studied 109 obese volunteers who underwent bariatric surgery, a procedure to remove parts of the stomach to induce weight loss. All the subjects lost weight, and three months after their surgery they demonstrated improved memory performance compared to a control group of obese volunteers who did not have the surgery.

Starve for Your Brain?

Researchers have explored whether calorie restriction might extend life expectancy and help keep the brain young. One of the leaders in this field from UCLA, Dr. Roy Walford, performed numerous animal studies demonstrating the health and longevity benefits of calorie restriction. He was so convinced of the validity of these findings that he began to fast, or starve himself, at least one day each week to protect his health. I remember seeing him eating light meals in the cafeteria on days when he *did* have lunch. He looked healthy but quite thin.

Fasting for even one day a week may be too stressful for the average person, and we don't yet know the ideal level of calorie restriction that might optimize health. Instead of fasting between large meals, many doctors and nutritionists advise people to eat several small meals throughout the day to help them maintain steady blood sugar levels and keep their appetite in check.

Although being obese or overweight appears to accelerate brain aging, some studies suggest that this may not be the case at certain times in our lives. Dr. Annette Fitzpatrick at the University of Washington and her associates studied nearly 2,800 middle-aged and older adults without dementia. They found that middle-age obesity increased the risk for developing dementia after five years, but *late-life* obesity was associated with a lower dementia risk. This "obesity paradox" may reflect the fact that weight loss in older people is linked to some age-related illnesses and can reflect poor general health. Unexplained weight loss is observed in patients who develop Alzheimer's disease, and it may predate the onset of dementia symptoms by as much as a decade.

As researchers try to answer the "to eat or not to eat" question, scientists at the University of California, San Francisco, have revealed how a low-carbohydrate/low-calorie diet, or a *ketogenic diet*, might delay the effects of aging on the brain. They found that a calorie-restricted ketogenic diet produces ketone bodies that provide the energy we need during fasting and exercise. These ketone bodies also protect us from oxidative stress that wears down and ages our cells.

No Rusty Brains

If you bought a new 10-speed bicycle for your son or grandson, you probably wouldn't like it if he left it out in the rain to rust. The rusting process is oxidation, which will eat away at the bike's shiny new chrome.

As brain cells perform their work, they generate by-products known as *free radicals*, and these free radicals cause a similar process of oxidative stress that wears away at our brains. Luckily, eating a healthy diet rich in antioxidant fruits and vegetables helps fight off this oxidative damage and protects our brains. The World Health Organization recommends having at least five servings of fruits and vegetables each day.

Although many older people do not eat enough antioxidant fruits and vegetables, our UCLA research with the Gallup Poll organization showed that on average, older people consume more fruits and vegetables than middle-aged or young adults. In a representative sample of 18,552 US respondents, 64 percent of older adults reported that they ate the recommended amount on four or more days in the previous week, compared with 54 percent of middle-aged people and 49 percent of young adults. And those who consumed more fruits and vegetables had significantly fewer memory complaints.

Fruits and vegetables with vibrant colors, such as blueberries, pomegranates, kale, and broccoli, are filled with polyphenol antioxidants. Eating these and other fruits and vegetables is associated with a lower risk for developing Alzheimer's disease and related forms of dementia.

Your specific daily need for fruits and vegetables depends on your total daily calorie intake. If you consume about 2,000

```
Examples of Antioxidant Fruits and Vegetables:
```

Fruits		Vegetables	
Avocados	Peaches	Alfalfa sprouts	Corn
Blackberries	Pears	Artichokes	Onions
Blueberries	Plums	Beets	Radishes
Cantaloupe	Pomegranates	Bell peppers	Romaine lettuce
Cherries	Prunes	Broccoli	Spinach
Cranberries	Raisins	Brussels sprouts	Sweet potatoes
Grapes	Raspberries	Cabbage	Swiss chard
Kiwifruit	Strawberries	Carrots	Turnip greens
Mango	Tomatoes	Cauliflower	Winter squash
Oranges		Kale	

calories a day, you should make two cups of fruits and two and a half cups of vegetables part of those calories. A piece of fruit such as a banana or apple is equivalent to a cup, as is a half cup of dried fruit. In addition to antioxidants, fruits and vegetables provide other vitamins, minerals, and fibers that protect the body and brain from accelerated aging. If you are watching your weight, keep in mind that dried fruits like prunes and raisins, though rich in antioxidants, are also high in calories.

Fruits and vegetables also contain phytonutrients, chemical compounds that protect plants from germs and bugs and are responsible for many of the odors and pigments in plant foods, such as the deep purple of blueberries and the strong smell of garlic. Nuts, whole grains, beans, herbs, spices, and tea also contain phytonutrients. Although they are not essential for keeping us alive like vitamins and minerals, phytonutrients do help maintain normal body functions and prevent some diseases. Phytonutrients such as the flavonoids in apples, berries, and onions are strong antioxidants. Preliminary studies indicate that the phytonutrient lycopene, found in tomatoes, pink grapefruit, watermelon, and guava, may protect against some forms of neurodegeneration and cancer.

Spice Is Nice for Your Brain

Most Americans have become used to foods that contain too much salt, which raises the risk for high blood pressure and other illnesses that threaten brain health. Better alternatives are herbs and spices, which add color and flavor to your food as well as brain-boosting antioxidants. So instead of reaching for the saltshaker, try some basil, cloves, chili powder, cinnamon, ginger, oregano, parsley, pepper, or turmeric (found in curry powder).

Eating Right Fights Brain Inflammation

Inflammation is a normal physiological process that protects our bodies from infection and helps us recover from injuries. If you sprain your ankle, it will swell, redden, hurt, and feel warm. Those are all signs that your inflammatory system is working to repair the injured tissue. With rest, the swelling and redness eventually resolve and you can walk free of pain again.

Research has led scientists to believe that an overly zealous inflammatory system may contribute to Alzheimer's disease, heart disease, and other age-related illnesses. It's possible to measure the level of inflammation in the body with a blood test. High levels of inflammation in the blood are associated with shorter life expectancy and higher risk of cardiac disease.

In studies of patients with Alzheimer's disease, inflammation has been detected throughout the brain, especially in regions that control thinking and memory. Chronic brain inflammation can make people forgetful and moody, and can contribute to symptoms of depression.

Several studies indicate that anti-inflammatory lifestyle strategies can lower the risk for Alzheimer's disease. Both daily cardiovascular exercise and getting a good night's sleep are believed to fight brain inflammation, as well as consuming foods that have anti-inflammatory effects.

Omega-3 fats are anti-inflammatory essential fatty acids that our bodies require to remain healthy. They are called essential because our bodies cannot produce them so we must get them from our diet. Omega-3 fatty acids are highly concentrated in the brain and critical to brain function, growth, and development. Also known as polyunsaturated fatty acids, or PUFAs, they can be consumed from fish, nuts, and some plant oils such as canola oil.

By reducing inflammation, omega-3 fatty acids help decrease the risk of arthritis, heart disease, cancer, and Alzheimer's disease. One important omega-3, docosahexaenoic acid, or DHA, is necessary for normal brain activity and protects against Alzheimer's-type toxins. High blood levels of DHA in middle-aged adults are associated with improved learning abilities and better performance scores on cognitive testing. Low levels of brain DHA are linked to age-related cognitive decline and greater risk for Alzheimer's disease.

Unfortunately, the typical American diet does not include enough omega-3 fats. We tend to ingest more omega-6 fats from whole milk, red meats, butter, fried foods, and certain vegetable oils like corn oil — all of which promote inflammation. Although we do need a small amount of omega-6 fat for normal brain development, muscle growth, and a healthy nervous system, the average American consumes 20 times more omega-6 fat than anti-inflammatory omega-3. The recommended ratio is closer to 3 to 1.

Eating fish and seafood is a great way to get omega-3 fats. It's a good idea to get fish caught in the wild as opposed to farmed

Coconut Oil and Alzheimer's Disease

Many people want to know whether coconut oil protects the brain from Alzheimer's disease. After consuming coconut oil, our bodies break down part of it into ketone bodies, which can provide an alternative source of energy for our brains along with glucose. Investigators at the University of South Florida Health Byrd Alzheimer's Institute are recruiting volunteers to determine if coconut oil is any better than an inactive placebo in protecting the brain from Alzheimer's disease. Until results from such systematic studies come in, the brain health benefits of coconut oil are still in question. Keep in mind that coconut oil is a saturated fat, which can increase risk for heart disease.

fish, because farmed fish contains more total fat and higher amounts of omega-6 fats. Most experts recommend eating fish no more than two or three times a week so that you don't consume excess mercury. Larger predatory fish like swordfish and shark have higher mercury concentrations than smaller fish like trout or catfish. To compare the mercury levels of different fish and seafood, visit the Monterey Bay Aquarium Seafood Watch site (www.seafoodwatch.org).

GOOD SOURCES OF OMEGA-3 FATS

Fish and seafood: Anchovies, cod, crab, herring, lobster, mackerel, salmon, sardines, scallops, trout, tuna

Beans: Kidney, mung, pinto

Nuts and seeds: Flaxseed, pecans, pine nuts, walnuts

Oils: Canola, flaxseed, cod liver, soybean

Eat Like a Mediterranean

When it comes to a brain-healthy diet, 65 million Frenchmen can't be wrong. Neither can 62 million Italians or 47 million Spaniards. Residents of these and other countries bordering the Mediterranean Sea share nutritional habits that not only protect heart health, they help keep brains young by reducing the risk for Alzheimer's disease and dementia.

The younger brain diet that I recommend is very much like a Mediterranean-style diet that emphasizes fruits, vegetables, nuts, legumes, whole grains, vegetable oils (especially olive oil), fish, and other lean proteins. By contrast, a typical North American diet emphasizes red meat and dairy products. Numerous studies have shown that people who adhere to a Mediterranean diet have a lower risk for age-related mental decline and Alzheimer's disease.

In a 2012 study of 966 older volunteers, Dr. Hannah Gardener and coworkers at the University of Miami found less evidence of

The Skinny on Omega-9 Fats

In addition to omega-3s, a Mediterranean-style diet includes omega-9 fatty acids from foods like olive oil, canola oil, peanuts, almonds, cashews, pistachios, avocados, and olives. Omega-9 fats are nonessential, meaning our bodies can manufacture them if necessary, so we don't need to take them as supplements, but dietary omega-9 fatty acids bolster body and brain health in several ways. Because these fats lower "bad" LDL cholesterol and increase "good" HDL cholesterol, they reduce stroke risk and boost cardiovascular health. Recent research also indicates that omega-9 fats help increase metabolism and improve mood. Although olive oil and butter contain comparable calories per tablespoon, substituting olive oil for butter may help us to control overall calorie intake. In a study of restaurant goers, Cornell University investigators found that people given olive oil with their bread ate 23 percent less bread compared with those given butter.

brain damage on MRI scans in people who consumed a Mediterranean diet. The MRI testing showed that eating this healthy diet was associated with less injury to the small blood vessels of the brain that service the white matter, which transmits signals from one brain cell to another.

Other studies have confirmed this type of diet's brain-protective benefits. Dr. Nikolaos Scarmeas and associates at Columbia University in New York followed 1,393 older research volunteers over a four and a half-year period. They found that participants who adhered to a Mediterranean-style diet were less likely to develop mild cognitive impairment or dementia. So whether you're dining in the South of France or preparing dinner at home, make sure to include anti-inflammatory omega-3 fatty acids from fish; healthy vitamins, minerals, and fibers from whole grains; plenty of antioxidant-rich fruits and vegetables; and healthy fats such as olive oil.

Big on Protein

A Mediterranean-style diet emphasizes healthy proteins from nuts and fish along with healthy carbohydrates from whole grains and antioxidant fruits and vegetables. Combining these two food groups — proteins and carbohydrates — is a key strategy for keeping your brain young. Carbohydrates alone provide an immediate energy boost, but that boost wanes after a short while. If I eat an apple at 10 in the morning, I may feel satisfied for an hour, but then I'm hungry again. If I had instead combined the apple (carbohydrates) with a handful of walnuts or a cup of yogurt (proteins), I would have gotten a quick energy lift from the carbs and enjoyed longer-lasting satiety from the proteins. Because healthy proteins make us feel full longer, they help control hunger and body weight.

It's not entirely clear how proteins curb appetite. One possibility is that protein lowers brain levels of appetite-stimulating hormones. Consuming protein may also lead to fewer spikes of insulin so that blood sugar levels remain constant. When blood sugar drops, appetite increases.

Proteins are critical to the structure and function of our bodies and brains. Protein molecules consist of 20 amino acid building blocks, nine of which are essential, so we must get them from our diet. Essential amino acids are present in fish, meat, poultry, yogurt, eggs, milk, cheese, nuts, and soybeans.

Some people consume a high-protein, low-carbohydrate diet in an effort to lose weight, but it's important to note that eating too much protein may be counterproductive. A diet consisting of 50 percent protein would not allow for enough healthy carbs

Full-Fat Yogurt Reduces Obesity Risk

A new study discounts the accepted wisdom of eating low-fat or nonfat yogurt to avoid weight gain. Professor Miguel Martinez-Gonzalez of the University of Navarra, Spain, presented the results of a six-year investigation of 8,516 volunteers who had a healthy weight at the start of the study. Those who consumed three and a half cups of full-fat yogurt each week were 19 percent less likely to become obese compared with those who ate low-fat or no yogurt at all. The weight-control benefits from full-fat yogurt were even greater for volunteers who also consumed a Mediterranean-style diet.

and could potentially be very high in fat. A 30 percent protein diet provides more protein than the average American diet (about 15 percent) and still leaves room for fruits, vegetables, and whole grains.

 SMART SNACK COMBINATIONS
- Walnuts and raisins
- Celery sticks with natural almond butter
- Sliced apple with string cheese
- Yogurt mixed with blueberries
- Sardines on whole-grain crackers

Refine Your Ideas on Sugars

Our brains require energy to function correctly, and they get that energy from glucose, a form of sugar that comes from eating carbohydrates. Because our brain cells can't store glucose, they need a steady supply from the bloodstream.

As sugar is consumed, the pancreas secretes insulin, the hormone that moves sugar from the blood to the body's cells. Foods that contain large amounts of refined or processed carbohydrates like cookies and white rice have a high glycemic index, meaning they cause large and rapid blood sugar spikes that increase insulin release. This increased insulin causes cells to absorb glucose too quickly. Over time, the cells become insulin resistant and require more and more of it to do their job.

People in the habit of eating high glycemic index foods have a heightened risk for diabetes. Consuming healthier low glycemic index foods such as fresh fruits, vegetables, and whole grains helps maintain steady blood sugar levels and allows insulin to function normally. To lower your risk for diabetes, eat low glycemic index foods.

The insulin resistance of diabetes threatens brain health — it interferes with glucose traveling from the blood to brain cells

---

Lab Animals Choose Oreos Over Cocaine

Have you ever tried to eat just one Oreo cookie and instead ended up devouring the rest of the package? Research indicates that this high-fat/high-sugar snack stimulates the brain's nucleus accumbens pleasure center in the same way that highly addictive drugs like cocaine do. In 2013, Dr. Joseph Schroeder and colleagues at Connecticut College reported that laboratory animals that raced their way through a maze to reach either Oreo cookies or cocaine spent significantly more time with the cookies than the drug. In fact, the Oreos activated the animals' nucleus accumbens more than the cocaine did. Many experts believe that these animal results are relevant to humans and help explain the highly addictive potential of high-fat/high-sugar foods. My advice to those who can't resist Oreos: take out one or two and stow the rest of the bag. Better yet, grab an orange instead.

---

and compromises the brain's main energy source. Diabetes also increases the risk for small strokes in the brain and for developing Alzheimer's disease.

Eating large amounts of refined sugar piles on extra calories that can lead to weight gain, and sugary drinks are a common source. Research has linked sugary drinks to obesity risk, so switching to water or tea can help people control body weight. A recent study published in the journal *BMC Public Health* showed that imposing a monetary tax on sugar-sweetened beverages could actually reduce obesity rates.

Caffeine and Alcohol

Caffeinated and alcoholic drinks are not just popular throughout the world; they are integral to many social interactions. The phrases "meet for coffee" or "how about a drink" are almost synonymous with "let's get together." The negative consequences of overindulging in either are well known. Too much coffee can make you anxious or jittery and even put your heart at risk. Alcoholism devastates lives as well as brain cells. Chronic alcohol abuse can destroy the hippocampal memory center of the brain and lead to profound amnesia. However, in moderation, these beverages have actually been associated with better brain health.

Caffeinated beverages help dilate blood vessels, making them work more effectively. Drinking one to three cups of coffee a day has been linked to a 65 percent lower risk for developing Alzheimer's and Parkinson's disease. Scientists have shown that when laboratory animals consume coffee every day, it protects their brain cells from the harmful effects of excess cholesterol. Researchers at the University of South Florida College of Pharmacy followed patients with mild cognitive impairment for several years and reported that those who progressed to dementia had caffeine blood levels 50 percent lower than those whose cognitive state remained stable.

Most of us have experienced the immediate effects of caffeine — it perks us up and makes us feel more alert and focused. A recent study of volunteers who were not habitual coffee drinkers showed significant memory improvements a full 24 hours after consuming one to two cups of coffee.

Some people get an upset stomach from coffee's acidity and other chemicals besides caffeine. A cup of tea can be an excellent substitute for them, but tea doesn't pack the same caffeine punch as coffee. A cup of brewed coffee contains 100 to 200 milligrams of caffeine compared to only about 40 milligrams in a cup of tea.

Moderate alcohol consumption is also believed to protect the brain. Light drinkers have about a 30 percent lower risk for dementia when compared to alcohol abstainers or those who drink in excess. People often wonder what "light" or "moderate" alcohol consumption means. Research suggests that one daily glass of spirits or wine for women and two glasses for men are in the brain-healthy range. This difference probably reflects the fact that men are usually larger than women and thus tolerate higher alcohol consumption.

Exactly why light alcohol consumption may protect the brain is still being determined. One theory is that people who drink

---

Eating for a Younger Brain

- Make your diet delicious and nutritious. In just two weeks, you can alter your brain's neural circuits and make it easier to stick with your diet and enjoy it.
- Some people can become addicted to certain foods or too much food, so it's important to recognize and avoid anything that might trigger you to overeat.
- Eat at least five servings of a variety of colorful fruits and vegetables every day to fight off your brain's oxidative stress.
- Omega-3 fats from fish, nuts, and flaxseed are natural anti-inflammatories and protect brain cells from age-related damage.
- Being overweight or obese is bad for your brain so if weight is a concern, limit your caloric intake and increase your activity level.
- Combining healthy proteins and carbohydrates at every meal and snack will boost your energy and keep you satisfied longer.
- Protect your brain by cutting back on refined sugars in your diet. This will lower your risk for becoming overweight or obese, and for developing diabetes.
- Caffeine and alcohol are good for your brain if consumed in moderation.

---

in moderation tend to live more moderate lifestyles in general, which may protect their brains because they don't overindulge in things. Some studies point to the potentially brain-protective chemicals in alcohol. Researchers at Mount Sinai School of Medicine in New York found that laboratory animals that ingest the mouse equivalent of a six-ounce glass of wine each day have better memory ability than control mice. They also have fewer of the amyloid plaques that are found in the brains of Alzheimer's victims.

Antioxidants in alcohol may also protect the brain. One of these antioxidant compounds, resveratrol, is abundant in grapes and wine, and animal studies have shown that resveratrol improves memory. But before you run out and stock up on brain-boosting resveratrol capsules, keep in mind that human studies are still ongoing.

CHAPTER SIX

Keep Fit for a Younger Brain

"The first time I see a jogger smiling, I'll consider it."
—*Joan Rivers*

H E HEARS THE EVEN beating of his heart as he glides across the ground, his limbs propelling him further and further in perfect alignment. The air is fresh and his mind is calm as he rounds the corner toward home. He slows his pace and walks up the driveway, glistening and happy. Greg loves his morning run.

Carolyn hands him a glass of orange juice and asks, "How many miles today?"

"Five. It was fantastic."

"Happy birthday, darling," she says, kissing him on his sweaty forehead. "You're 73 years young."

We know that aerobic conditioning helps maintain physical health. Greg's daily run lowers his risk for diabetes and heart disease and extends his life expectancy. Recent research shows that physical exercise is also one of the most powerful ways to keep our brains young, reduce risk of dementia, and even take years off our brain age.

Getting up off the couch and walking, gardening, or doing any physical activity that makes your heart pump more oxygen and nutrients to your brain cells pays off in immediate mental improvements. Scientists have documented the short-term cognitive benefits of exercise: it increases our ability to focus attention, solve problems, and plan the future — mental abilities necessary to function well in everyday life.

Physical exercise produces an extraordinary chemical that functions as a neuron activator — brain-derived neurotrophic factor, or BDNF. This chemical repairs damaged brain cells and stimulates healthy ones to sprout more branches for better neural communication and brain performance. A 2013 study published in the *Journal of the American Medical Association Neurology* found that volunteers with high levels of BDNF in the blood had about half the likelihood of developing dementia after 10 years of follow-up.

Working out also lifts our mood. Physical exercise bathes our brains with endorphins, the "feel good" hormones responsible for the euphoria that many long-distance runners and other endurance athletes report. Remaining consistently active has been linked to better life satisfaction, psychological well-being, and fewer symptoms of depression.

Studies have found that the mood-lifting effect of exercise is comparable to that of antidepressants for mild to moderate depression. Maintaining a good mood has been shown to improve cognitive performance and is associated with a lower risk for developing dementia and Alzheimer's disease.

Exercise at Every Age

Greg had been a runner since high school. Even in his 70s, people still told him he looked 10 years younger, and he felt that way too. The earlier in life one begins an exercise habit, the easier it is to continue that healthy habit over the years, but it's never too late to get started.

New studies indicate that young people who live sedentary lifestyles pay the price later. Dr. Kristine Yaffe and associates from the University of California, San Francisco, recently reported that middle-aged people have better cognitive abilities if they were active as young adults. The investigators analyzed data from a 25-year longitudinal study that included 3,375 middle-aged volunteers from four US cities. They found that those who engaged in more exercise in their youth performed better on cognitive tests for speed of mental processing and executive functioning — both of which directly affect thinking and problem solving.

Exercising bolsters brain health at every age, and numerous studies have shown that physical fitness in older adults produces immediate and long-term positive brain effects. Middle-aged people who take up exercise lower their risk for developing dementia later. Investigators at the University of California, Irvine, found that 90-year-olds in good physical condition (e.g., stronger grip, better balance) are less likely to experience memory loss and other forms of cognitive decline.

Exercise Makes Your Brain Bigger

Exercise can actually make your brain bigger, and a bigger brain is a better brain. Landmark studies performed by Dr. Arthur Kramer and coworkers at the University of Illinois demonstrated that physically fit older volunteers had better memory abilities and bigger hippocampal memory centers when compared to those who were inactive.

The scientists studied 120 volunteers between ages 60 and 80. Half began a brisk walking program that involved wearing heart rate monitors that encouraged them to walk at their target heart rate zone, while the other half did only stretching and toning exercises. MRI brain scans, blood tests, and memory assessments were performed on both groups before they began (baseline) and after six and 12 months.

The chart below shows the volumes of the volunteers' left hippocampus, a horseshoe-shaped brain area situated beneath the temples, which stores and organizes new verbal memories so they can be retrieved later. In the aerobic exercise group, the left hippocampus grew steadily, while it gradually shrank in the group that only stretched and toned. The same pattern was documented in the right hippocampus, which controls visual and spatial memory.

The aerobic training increased the size of the overall hippocampus by two percent, effectively reversing age-related volume loss by two years. The scientists also found that enlargement of this memory center was associated with better memory performance scores and higher blood levels of BDNF, the chemical that stimulates nerve cell growth in the brain.

The volunteers who walked gradually increased their pace over the first seven weeks of the study. This strategy helped them boost their cardiovascular stamina and their lower extremity strength, which is helpful for avoiding exhaustion, soreness, and injury. If you are not in shape, it's a good idea to begin exercising

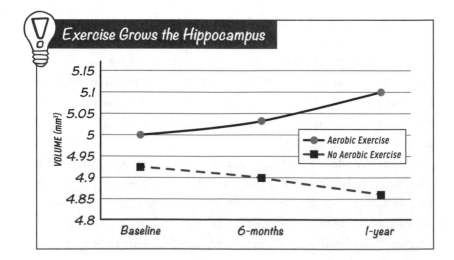

slowly and steadily, increasing your pace and duration as your endurance grows. Sporadic exercisers or weekend warriors do get occasional workouts, but they don't have the opportunity to build up their stamina and are at greater risk for injury.

WALK TO BEAT DIABETES

A regular exercise routine not only boosts brain function, it also protects your body from diabetes, a common age-related illness that afflicts 26 million Americans. Just 20 minutes a day of brisk walking can cut your risk for diabetes by as much as 30 percent. Your brain will benefit too, since having diabetes doubles your risk for Alzheimer's.

Christy had been noticing subtle memory slips for years but kidded around about it like the rest of her friends did. After reading a convincing article about how physical exercise could improve memory, she decided to get physically active again to help her memory. Unfortunately, Christy didn't bother to gauge her baseline first.

She had been an athlete in high school and college and still had her track and volleyball trophies to prove it. But after graduating, she got too busy with her job and raising a family to continue exercising.

Now Christy wanted to dive right in again. She decided to skip her Saturday morning errands and make that her workout time. She woke up early, got dressed, tore out the front door, and jogged up the steep slope of her street. The fresh air felt great and although she got a bit winded after a couple of minutes, she managed to push through it. She did feel a slight twinge in her right knee going up the last hill, but she knew it was downhill from there. Unfortunately, running downhill made her knee feel worse.

After just 20 minutes, Christy's knee was throbbing. She limped back into the house, grabbed an icepack for her knee, and took some aspirin. She was forced to accept the fact that at 57, she didn't have the stamina or the knees she had at 20.

Christy got some physical therapy to help heal her knee, and after a month she could walk without pain again. She found a trainer to help her create a reasonable exercise routine that would build up her stamina gradually from her current fitness level. Pretty soon working out felt terrific, just like it had in school, but now she got an added benefit — an improved memory.

Gauge Your Baseline Fitness

Whether we enjoy walking, jogging, playing tennis, or briskly operating a remote control while relaxing on the couch, we all have a current or baseline physical fitness level. Knowing our baseline helps us determine where to begin our physical exercise program. It reveals our existing physical strengths and limitations.

Studies have shown that just self-rating our own fitness level can give us a pretty good idea of what our actual performance scores will be. To help get a sense of your current level of fitness, complete this brief questionnaire to self-assess your cardiovascular conditioning, strength levels, and coordination abilities. The numerical scores will clue you into how much to focus on each area when you begin your 2-Week Younger Brain Program.

If you scored 4 to 6 in each category, you are in pretty good physical shape. If your scores are higher than 8 in any of the three categories, then you have some work to do. Your efforts will be an important investment in your brain and body health, and you'll notice results quickly. Just as Christy did with her trainer, you should start exercising at your current fitness level and gradually build up your workout routine to obtain optimal benefits.

Make Exercise Fun

In America, two out of every five people are completely sedentary, and rates of inactivity increase with age. Many people not only have difficulty making time for exercise, they have trouble

Your Baseline Physical Fitness

Indicate below the degree to which you agree with the statements by circling a number: 1 (never), 2 (sometimes), or 3 (usually).

Cardiovascular Conditioning	Never	Somtimes	Usually
I am out of breath after a brisk 10-minute walk.	1	2	3
I get tired after climbing two flights of stairs.	1	2	3
I usually take the elevator instead of the stairs.	1	2	3
I lag behind others when walking or hiking.	1	2	3
Total Cardiovascular Score	___	___	___

Strength Levels	Never	Somtimes	Usually
I get tired standing in line for more than 10 minutes.	1	2	3
I ask others to lift heavy objects for me.	1	2	3
It is hard for me to open a tight jar or window.	1	2	3
I feel sore after trying new sports or physical activities	1	2	3
Total Strength Score	___	___	___

Coordination Abilities	Never	Somtimes	Usually
I worry about tripping or falling while walking.	1	2	3
I cannot stand on one leg for more than five seconds.	1	2	3
I have to sit down to put on shoes.	1	2	3
I need a handrail or assistance on stairs.	1	2	3
Total Coordination Score	___	___	___

finding any fun in it. If you create an exercise routine that you enjoy, like walking with friends, playing tennis with a good partner, or taking a fun Zumba class at the gym, it's easier to stick with it.

The brain-protective effects of exercise have been documented in multiple studies, and they indicate that sporadic exercise is not enough to really benefit the brain. We need to continue exercising for months and years in order to delay the onset of debilitating forms of brain aging, such as dementia and Alzheimer's disease.

Dr. Thorleif Etgen and colleagues at the Technical University of Munich studied the cognitive effects of physical activity in nearly 4,000 people aged 55 and older. Those who exercised routinely over a two-year period lowered their risk for developing cognitive decline by approximately 50 percent compared to those who remained inactive. You don't have to become a triathlete to reduce your risk for dementia; you just need to stick with an exercise program for the long haul. Dr. Eric Larson and associates at the University of Washington followed volunteers over six years and found that exercising just three days a week led to significantly lower risks for dementia in people age 65 and older.

When we get a really good workout, our bodies produce endorphins — natural analgesics that lift our mood and reinforce the experience. Our brain's dopamine system gets charged up, rewarding us for breaking a sweat, and our brain starts to crave more exercise.

Five Tips to Make Exercise Fun

1. **Make it social.** Enjoying conversation while working out with friends benefits both your body and your brain.

2. **Compete.** The heated excitement of tennis, volleyball, and other competitive sports engages our brains and keeps us coming back. If you'd prefer not to compete against others, compete against yourself by continually challenging yourself to improve your times or increase your number of repetitions.

3. **Add brain games.** Do puzzles and brain teasers while on the stationary bike or treadmill: new research shows that you get more out of mental workouts when your heart is pumping hard at the same time.

4. **Shake it up.** Your brain loves variety, so don't just stick with one routine or sport.

5. **Get outdoors.** Swap the treadmill for the outdoors sometimes so you can enjoy the scenery and explore new surroundings while you exercise.

Many people prefer exercising in the morning, while others find it more convenient later in the day. The key is to exercise when you feel the most energetic. When you exercise regularly your mind and body will begin to look forward to your workout, and soon it will become a habit. Scientists who study habit formation have found that for many individuals, new behaviors can transform into regular habits in just three weeks. However, there are exceptions and some people may need a month or longer to turn their exercise routine into a habit.

WORLD'S OLDEST MARATHON RUNNER

On October 16, 2011, Fauja Singh became the oldest person to complete a marathon. At 100 years of age, Singh completed the 26-mile Toronto Waterfront Marathon in eight hours. It's never too late to start running marathons. Singh ran his first one at age 89.

People with good self-esteem and who perceive themselves as healthy are usually more motivated to continue exercising throughout their lives. Dr. Catherine Sarkisian's work at UCLA showed that when older adults are aware of the brain health and memory benefits of their exercise program, they are more likely to remain consistent with it.

When planning your exercise routine, it often helps to think back on what physical activities you enjoyed earlier in your life. Many people find competitive sports the most fun, while others prefer to challenge themselves by walking, jogging, swimming, or weight lifting.

No matter your sport of choice, cross-training by doing several different types of exercise is an important part of any fitness routine. Cross-training allows you to use your muscles differently, reduces your risk for injury, and keeps your workouts fun and interesting. For example, a marathon runner must practice long-distance running to excel, but lifting weights for increased strength and taking yoga for better flexibility will improve that runner's overall physical conditioning.

In the 2-Week Younger Brain Program, a daily exercise routine will be integrated with other brain health strategies, but there is no reason to wait until you read chapter 9. Why not start exercising right now?

EXERCISE BRAIN TEASER

Unscramble the letters below to find the exercise that focuses more on strength training than aerobic conditioning. (Answer at end of chapter.)

GOJNGGI   USPPHUS   MGMSINWI   AKLGINW   CCLINGY

Adapt for Injuries and Minimize Pain

Many of us feel better all over after a good workout. Neuroscientists have found that elevations in endorphin levels explain this analgesic effect and have pinpointed the areas of the brain that are affected by exercise. To experience this natural endorphin pain relief, our workouts need to get our hearts pumping fast enough to increase the oxygen and blood flow to our brains — a leisurely stroll to the corner newsstand may not always do the trick. Aerobic exercise also increases other neurotransmitters that can help alleviate pain, such as GABA (gamma amino butyric acid), which calms down the nervous system and makes us less susceptible to painful stimuli.

Most of us have no excuse for not exercising and enjoying the benefits of fitness through middle age and beyond. We can all adapt our exercise program to meet our personal needs and accommodate any prior injuries or age-related physical declines.

Many exercises can strengthen weak or injured areas of our bodies. People who suffer from knee or ankle issues may prefer the circular movements of an elliptical machine or bicycle, which are easier on those joints than jogging or running. Middle

Three Stretches At The Desk

Many of us spend hours each day sitting at a desk. Whether we're working with a computer, sorting mail, or balancing a checkbook, we tend to slouch our shoulders forward, round our backs, and hold our arms in the same position for long periods. It is important to stretch our muscles at regular intervals in order to maintain good posture and balance. Try these three stretches you can do without even standing up.

Chest — Sit at the edge of your seat, clasp your hands behind your back, and raise your straight arms out behind you, pushing your chest forward. Hold for five seconds and repeat. Feel your chest stretching and your shoulders opening up.

Triceps — Raise your arms over your head. Bend your right elbow, dropping your right hand behind your head. Clasp the bent right elbow with your left hand and pull it down and back behind your head. Hold for a count of five. Feel the stretch in your right triceps muscle and shoulder. Repeat with the other arm.

Shoulders — Reach one straight arm across your chest toward the other shoulder. With the opposite hand, grasp your elbow and pull that straight arm in closer to your chest. Feel the stretch in the front of your shoulder and your upper back. Hold for a count of five then repeat on the other side.

and lower back pain sufferers may fare better with the smooth, consistent movements of swimming that stretch and strengthen weak back muscles, rather than the jarring twists and turns of tennis or golf.

A good trainer or physical therapist can recommend specific corrective exercises to address muscle imbalances that may lead to chronic problems like back or knee pain. These corrective exercises are designed to improve movement and take you to the next level of your fitness training.

Protect Your Head

One of the downsides of some fun and engaging forms of exercise is the risk of head trauma or brain injury. Many professional athletes have suffered long-term consequences of repeated head injuries, but the dangers of traumatic brain injury are a concern for us all. The Centers for Disease Control and Prevention (CDC) recognizes the seriousness of the problem and

Symptoms of Concussion		
Dizziness	Vomiting	Unconsciousness
Headache	Vision changes	Depression
Confusion	Malaise	
Nausea	Muscle weakness	*If you suffer a blow to the*
Memory loss	Gait instability	*head, you should report*
Fatigue	Personality changes	*any symptoms to your*
Hearing loss	Irritability	*doctor immediately.*

estimates that at least 1.7 million traumatic brain injuries occur every year. Any sport that involves physical contact with an object or another person can lead to head trauma and concussion, including football, hockey, boxing, martial arts, soccer, cycling, skateboarding, and skiing.

Symptoms of concussion are varied and can include unconsciousness, headache, dizziness, nausea, vomiting, and fatigue. Repeated blows to the head, even those that do not cause a concussion, can lead to a condition known as chronic traumatic encephalopathy, or CTE, a syndrome that can alter personality, cause behavior and mood disturbances, and bring on symptoms including memory loss, confusion, dementia, depression, irritability, and suicidal behavior. Autopsies on the brains of patients who had CTE show high concentrations of tau, an abnormal protein deposit that is also found in brains of Alzheimer's disease victims.

Our UCLA research group has performed FDDNP-PET scans on retired National Football League players who reported CTE-like symptoms. In all the subjects, our studies showed high concentrations of FDDNP, indicating abnormally high amounts of tau protein in the same brain areas where tau was identified in autopsy studies of CTE patients. The amygdala, a region of the brain that controls emotion, displayed consistently high FDDNP signals. This may explain why patients with CTE experience irritability, impulsiveness, and other mood symptoms. These scans differed from typical Alzheimer's disease scans, but professional football players were found to have a significantly higher risk of developing Alzheimer's disease than the rest of us.

We are currently performing additional studies to learn if FDDNP-PET can help in early detection of traumatic brain injury. We suspect that although tau buildup is important, it is not the sole factor contributing to CTE symptoms. Genetic predisposition likely impacts CTE just as it does Alzheimer's disease. In fact, studies of career boxers have found that those with the APOE-4 Alzheimer's genetic risk are more likely to develop cognitive losses than those without it. Also, previous studies found that a traumatic brain injury early in life increases the risk for dementia in later life from twofold to fourfold when compared to the general population.

People don't always experience symptoms immediately after a traumatic brain injury, but that doesn't rule out bleeding or swelling in the brain that could be emerging silently. Following a blow to the head, it is essential to rest, avoid further injury, and seek medical attention.

In a Mayo Clinic study of 141 people with mild cognitive impairment (MCI), a pre-dementia condition, investigators found that nearly 20 percent of them had a history of one or more prior brain injuries. Brain scans of this 20 percent showed evidence of Alzheimer's disease, while study volunteers who had not experienced head trauma showed no evidence of the disease.

Wearing a helmet is necessary for many sports, including cycling and skateboarding. To protect your brain from injury, consider ways to make risky sports safer. Instead of riding your bike on a busy street, you might try riding a stationary bicycle at home — you can read or watch the news while you work out and protect your head at the same time. Tai chi is a gentler version of karate, and swimming laps is usually a safer alternative to surfing.

SAFER SPORTS ALTERNATIVES

Riskier Sport	Safer Sport
Surfing	Swimming
Tackle football	Touch or flag football
Mountain biking	Stationary bicycle
Helicopter skiing	Watching it on TV while on the treadmill

Fine-Tuning Your Workout

A complete fitness program covers all three vital areas: cardiovascular conditioning, strength training, and balance work. When planning your routine, it helps to try different forms of exercise for each area; you may discover you love tennis but find jogging boring. Also, some types of workouts will suit your lifestyle better than others, like using an indoor elliptical machine versus hiking outdoors. A program designed to match your personal tastes and needs will be easier to stick with for the long run.

Changing up your routine has advantages as well. It will make your workouts more interesting, and your brain will like it too. Numerous studies have shown that our brains are hardwired to seek novelty and explore new experiences, so alternating the types of exercise you do not only improves your overall fitness, it keeps your neural circuits happy.

Although all three fitness areas are important, the aerobic component is the most essential for your brain and heart health. It quickly improves your mood, mental acuity, energy levels, and sleep patterns. On days when you just can't set aside 15 or 20 minutes for some kind of aerobic exercise, try taking the stairs instead of the elevator and opt for walking between errands and appointments as much as possible during the day.

Setting goals can help motivate you to exercise, but make those goals realistic and attainable — increase the duration of your workouts by 5 minutes rather than 30 minutes at a time.

> ### Target Heart Rates
>
> Wearing a heart-rate monitor on your wrist can help you build your endurance to-
> ward a target heart rate and help you maintain that target rate when you reach
> it. You can calculate your maximum heart rate by subtracting your age from 220.
> The average 60-year-old has a maximum heart rate of 160 (220–60). Your workout
> target rate should not be your maximum heart rate but somewhere between 60 and
> 80 percent of it. So a 60-year-old should set and maintain a target heart-rate range
> of 96 to 128 during her cardiovascular exercise session.

Many people like to wear pedometers or heart monitors to see when they've reached their goals. Using these measuring methods is both effective and safe.

Aerobic Fitness Options

The aim of aerobic exercise is to get your heart and lungs to efficiently pump oxygen and nutrients to your brain cells. With greater cardiac efficiency, your body and brain also benefit from a lower risk for high blood pressure, diabetes, and other age-related diseases that can damage neurons. Burning calories while doing aerobic exercises also helps control excess body weight, which further optimizes brain health.

Some trainers tout the advantages of interval training, or interspersing low-intensity and high-intensity exercises, with brief rest periods in between. When interval training was compared to regular continuous training, both demonstrated similar increases in blood flow and heart and lung function. You can also split your exercise session into several brief periods if your schedule requires. Research has shown that dividing a 30-minute workout into three 10-minute sessions yields similar weight control and heart health benefits as doing a 30-minute routine straight through.

Walking has received the greatest attention in studies of aerobic conditioning because it has the lowest risk for injury, and

Walking and Creativity

You may have noticed that some of your most creative ideas don't always occur to you while working at your desk, but instead they come while you're outside taking a walk. Researchers at Stanford University assessed whether there is a real connection between exercise and creativity. They used a standard creativity test that asks subjects to come up with different ways to use common objects. The subjects demonstrated greater creativity while walking outside or on a treadmill than when seated at a desk, suggesting that the physiological effects of aerobic exercise may be stimulating neural circuits that control creative thinking. The next time I get writer's block, I'm going to take a walk.

most experts agree that walking delivers the same benefits as any other form of cardiovascular exercise.

Using a treadmill can be convenient, but it is slightly easier than walking or running outside because it lacks the air resistance of the outdoors. Increasing your walking pace to a jog or run will further push you toward your exercise goals, and adding a slight incline to your treadmill will increase the challenge of your indoor workout.

Finding an exercise buddy or group of friends to work out with can help keep us on a regular fitness schedule. Walking the dog is also a great excuse to get outside and get a brisk aerobic workout. Research indicates that having to walk the dog is an effective motivation for daily exercise. Investigators found that dog owners were more likely to take walks and lost more weight over a 50-week period than people without pets. And as an added benefit, your dog will stay in shape too.

Cycling is an effective aerobic option that is easy on the knees and ankles; in fact, the smooth circular movements actually strengthen those joints. If weather doesn't permit outdoor biking, stationary bikes or elliptical machines are great alternatives. Cycling builds up calf and thigh strength even more than walking or running, and it poses less risk of injury.

Swimming is an excellent low-impact exercise that engages nearly every major muscle group in the body. It benefits people with a variety of joint injuries, and varying your strokes helps facilitate healing. Swimming not only provides an aerobic workout, it can build muscle mass as well. A recent study found that older adults who swam regularly had better cardiorespiratory fitness and higher cognitive performance scores.

Racquet sports like tennis offer the fun of competition, which often motivates people to stay active, and the game's mental challenge provides cognitive benefits. The aerobic conditioning from tennis lowers body fat, cholesterol, and rates of cardiovascular disease and improves bone health. It also improves hand-eye coordination, movement, and balance. Less strenuous racquet sports, such as ping-pong, also provide these cognitive benefits.

Dancing, another great form of aerobic exercise, stimulates neural circuits in brain regions involved in motor control, balance, and social interaction. Brain scans of experienced dancers demonstrate greater ability in these brain functions compared to scans of novice dancers. But even the novice dancers have improved brainpower. A study of older novice dancers demonstrated superior cognitive, motor, and perceptual skills when compared with nondancers.

Household chores not only keep your home in order, they boost your heart rate and brain health. The physical benefits of housekeeping were highlighted by a Harvard study demonstrating lower body weight, blood pressure, and body mass index in Boston hotel maids who were told that their work satisfied the surgeon general's recommendations for an active lifestyle. Just knowing about the benefits of their work had a real impact on their health. Working around the house is a healthy form of physical conditioning for all of us. Raking leaves for 30 minutes can burn more than 200 calories, and a half hour of making beds can knock off about another 100.

Shopping at the mall may be hard on your credit card, but whether you're a big spender or an avid bargain hunter, you will benefit from the cardiovascular exercise you get briskly walking between stores and the neural stimulation that comes from searching through items for the right sizes and colors. Shopping activates brain regions that control memory, planning, and visual and spatial skills, as well as the neural circuits involved in social interactions and the fun of getting new things.

Of course, too much shopping can lead to financial stress, which has negative brain effects, but buyer's remorse can motivate some shoppers to go back to the stores to return items and reap the brain health benefits of navigating the mall again.

Strength Training: Building Muscle and Brain Bulk

Although aerobic exercise is essential for keeping our brains young, new scientific evidence highlights the additional benefits of strength training. Dumbbells and weight-lifting machines are not just for 20-somethings; middle-agers and seniors — even those 80 and older — can boost their brainpower by pumping iron on a regular basis. Strength training can take the form of resistance exercises using an elastic band or working out with free weights and machines. This type of exercise makes our bones denser, which is critically important for all of us as we age. Increased bone density lowers the risk for osteoporosis, which can lead to fractures from even minor falls. Strength training also stabilizes blood sugar, which lowers the risk for diabetes and its brain-aging consequences.

Workout with a Chair

You won't need a tennis court or gym for this exercise, which strengthens your hips, thighs, knees, calves, and lower back. It can even provide a nice aerobic boost. Sit at the edge of a chair with your back straight and feet shoulder-width apart. Place your hands behind your head with your chest forward and shoulders back. Slowly stand up straight and then gradually sit back down, pushing your bottom back behind you until it taps the chair. When it does, stand back up and repeat four times. Gradually increase your repetitions until you reach 20.

> ### Accessory-Free Isometrics
>
> Isometric strength-training exercises can be done with no bands, machines, or weights. They involve muscular contractions using your own body resistance. Try this isometric position to strengthen your upper body muscles (biceps, triceps, and chest). Place your palms against each other in front of your chest like someone who is praying and push them together as hard as you can. Hold the position for five seconds, rest, and repeat three times.

Strength training has been shown to elevate mood. Investigators randomly assigned 91 depressed patients to one hour of either aerobic exercise or strength training, three days a week. As predicted, oxygen use increased in the aerobic group and not in the strength-training group, but symptoms of depression improved in both groups. Other studies found that combining aerobic and strength training improves cognitive abilities in patients who have suffered a stroke.

A study of laboratory animals given strength-training exercises by attaching weights to their tails resulted in better performance on memory tests. The animals also had higher levels of a protein that resembles insulin and promotes brain cell growth.

Dr. Teresa Liu-Ambrose and colleagues at the University of British Columbia showed that weight training improves memory abilities in older women with mild cognitive impairment. They found that after six months of strength training, the women performed better on multiple cognitive tests compared to women who did no exercise. Their studies also indicated that aerobic and strength training may target different brain regions. Although strength training improved spatial memory skills in all the women, those who also engaged in aerobic exercise showed improved verbal memory scores as well.

Many trainers agree that strength training should involve working opposing muscle groups, such as biceps and triceps, to reduce the risk of injury. Doing a *split routine*, or building different muscle groups on alternate days, allows you to focus more on the specific muscles you are training that day, and it gives each muscle group a chance to rest and repair between sessions. Some weight trainers focus on upper body muscles (arms, shoulders, back, and chest) Monday, Wednesday, and Friday, leaving Tuesday, Thursday, and Saturday for lower-body workouts (thighs, calves, and hamstrings). On Sundays, many people get their exercise at the mall like my wife, Gigi.

When we think of strength training, many of us imagine gyms full of large weight machines, but there are other options:

Free weights allow you to strengthen specific muscle groups in a functional manner, meaning the exercises mimic the movements we make in real life. While weight machines can help beginners build strength, endurance, and good posture, free weights do the same but allow more variety of movement. If you've never used free weights, it may be a good idea to start with an experienced trainer who can show you the proper form to optimize the exercises and avoid injury. The American Heart Association and American College of Sports Medicine recommend that older adults work out their major muscle groups two or more nonconsecutive days each week.

Try These Resistance Band Exercises

1. **Bicep Curl.** Stand on the center of your band and grip the ends in each hand, palms facing forward. Keeping your elbows pinned against your sides, curl your lower arms up until your fists approach your shoulders. Now, slowly release your forearms back down to your sides. Repeat 4 to 10 times
2. **Upper Body Pull-Down.** Gripping both ends of your resistance band, stand with your feet wider than your shoulders and your toes pointing out. Raise your arms overhead and move them outward to form a V, pulling the band taut. Stretch the band even wider as you pull it down in front of your chest. Hold for a second and repeat three times. Gradually increase your repetitions as you get stronger.

Isolation exercises with resistance bands utilize elastic bands or straps that can be purchased at most drugstores and sporting goods stores. The color of the band usually indicates its resistance level. It's a good idea to start with an easy level and, as you build your strength, you can wrap or double up your band or move to a more difficult one to increase the resistance. The bands are easy to pack in a suitcase so they are great for travelers.

Maintaining Balance

Although a good sense of balance is vital for people at any age, it becomes especially important as we get older and have a higher risk of injury from falls. Investigators in the Netherlands gave 116 volleyball players a 36-week balance-training program. Afterward, they had significantly fewer ankle sprains when compared to a control group

Maintaining good balance is also an important mental task, which becomes more difficult as we age due to normal cognitive decline. Research has found that when older volunteers are given both cognitive and balance tasks simultaneously, they display much worse balance abilities than when they are given just a balance test alone.

We need a good sense of balance just to stand up straight. Our brain sends instant messages to our body to right itself if we become unstable, and it informs our muscle groups how much to work to keep us upright. Training in balance and stability frees up our minds to focus on other cognitive tasks.

 THE FLAMINGO
To perform this balance exercise, stand and focus on a point in front of you. Lift your right foot off the floor and use your outstretched arms to help you balance. Hold for a count of five and then switch to the other foot. Build up your stability level by holding the stance for an additional five seconds, gradually

increasing your time to 30 seconds on each leg. To challenge
yourself further, try this exercise with your eyes closed.

Tai chi is a popular exercise technique that involves slow,
smooth movements that provide several physical and mental
benefits. In addition to increasing balance and stability, it has
been shown to improve mood and lower stress levels. Studies of older adults who perform tai chi have shown that it can
improve their cognitive performance. Tai chi's brain health
benefits may result from improved blood flow, reduced inflammation, and increased levels of BDNF and other neuron
growth stimulants.

Pilates is an exercise method that increases strength, flexibility, and coordination. It focuses on strengthening and toning
the body's core muscle groups in the torso, including the abdomen, back, and hip muscles, which provide structural support
for our bodies and help maintain balance. In a recent study, attending a Pilates class two times a week was shown to improve
balance and posture after three months. To get started, consider hiring an instructor or joining a class because the standard
equipment is large and requires instruction to use. There are
also floor Pilates exercises that can be done anywhere with little
or no equipment.

Balance balls and boards are helpful for balance and stability training, stretching, and strengthening core muscles. This
inexpensive equipment helps us strengthen muscle groups that

 Pull-Down With Squat

Stand with your feet wider than your shoulders and your toes pointing out. Gripping
both ends of your resistance band, raise your arms overhead and move them outward
to form a V, pulling the band taut. As you bring the band down in front of your chest,
bend your knees and lower into a wide squat. As you return to standing, raise the
band back up above your head. Repeat five times. Gradually increase your repetitions.

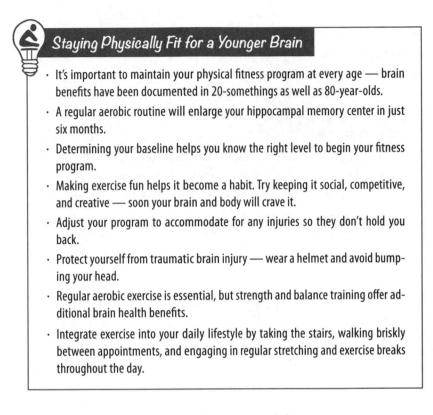

Staying Physically Fit for a Younger Brain

- It's important to maintain your physical fitness program at every age — brain benefits have been documented in 20-somethings as well as 80-year-olds.
- A regular aerobic routine will enlarge your hippocampal memory center in just six months.
- Determining your baseline helps you know the right level to begin your fitness program.
- Making exercise fun helps it become a habit. Try keeping it social, competitive, and creative — soon your brain and body will crave it.
- Adjust your program to accommodate for any injuries so they don't hold you back.
- Protect yourself from traumatic brain injury — wear a helmet and avoid bumping your head.
- Regular aerobic exercise is essential, but strength and balance training offer additional brain health benefits.
- Integrate exercise into your daily lifestyle by taking the stairs, walking briskly between appointments, and engaging in regular stretching and exercise breaks throughout the day.

maintain balance by introducing instability into any exercise, including push-ups and sit-ups. Scientists at Bond University in Australia reported that balance ball training led to significant benefits in lower back muscle endurance and flexibility, as well as leg strength and balance.

Yoga is an ancient practice that involves postures, breathing exercises, and meditation and provides cardiovascular and strength-training benefits. Scientists have begun to show how this form of exercise helps keep our brains young and healthy. A recent study assessed the impact of yoga on the brain's hippocampal memory center. Seven older healthy volunteers attended a regular yoga class for six months, after which their hippocampal memory centers were significantly larger. Another study found that the size of the brain's grey matter (the outer rim of the brain that contains neural cell bodies) was larger in people who practiced yoga for approximately five years compared with control subjects. The yoga practitioners also demonstrated better cognitive performance.

ANSWER TO EXERCISE BRAIN TEASER
Page 136:

If you correctly unscrambled the four words, you'd see that the second word, PUSHUPS, is the correct answer, since JOGGING, SWIMMING, WALKING, and CYCLING are all forms of aerobic conditioning.

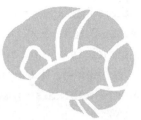

CHAPTER SEVEN

Good Friends Make Happy Neurons

"Outside of a dog, a book is man's best friend. Inside of a dog it's too dark to read."

—*Groucho Marx*

WHEN I LEFT LOS Angeles to do a residency across the country, I knew very few people in my new city. It took me a while to develop friendships and create a new social network, but once I did, I felt happier and more productive. I hadn't even realized that I had felt lonely until I made new friends.

Maintaining close relationships with other people is a basic human need. Interacting with family and friends not only increases our life expectancy, it lowers our risk for future cognitive decline by keeping our brains engaged and young. Spending time with colleagues at work also protects our brains. A French study of nearly half a million people showed that delaying retirement by just a few years will reduce the risk for Alzheimer's disease: someone who retires at age 65 has a 15 percent lower risk of developing dementia than someone who retires at 60.

Connecting with others affects our mind and body health. Our heart rate may accelerate and we may experience loving feelings when hugging a close friend or kissing a loved one. Social bonding and feelings of belonging increase the release of oxytocin, one of the brain's most powerful feel-good hormones.

Disengaging from your usual social ties is not good for your mind health: prolonged isolation can actually drive people crazy. Prisoners in solitary confinement or experimental subjects exposed to extended periods of solitude can develop full-blown psychosis with hallucinations and delusions. The mind is pushed to create fantasy relationships when deprived of real ones.

Our experience of close human contact shapes our brain development from infancy. Babies who have been adequately nourished but not held or caressed by their mothers often experience developmental delays. Seclusion and neglect early in life can lead to future emotional problems and cognitive impairments. Recent research indicates that early isolation slows

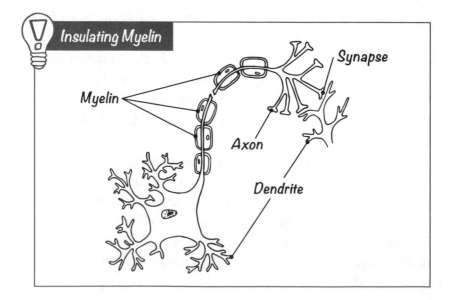

down the communication between developing brain regions by impeding the growth of myelin, which insulates neuronal connections — the long wires between neurons that are critical to learning.

This insulating myelin, contained in the brain's white matter, allows for transmission of electrical signals at synapses, or the gaps where one cell's axon (the long transmitting brain wire) meets the next cell's dendrite (the shorter receiving end). Without sufficient myelin insulation, these currents of electric signal will leak outside the cells and slow down the communication between one nerve cell and the next. Thin or damaged myelin leads to impaired thinking and memory loss.

Children who have suffered from neglect have less white matter myelin in their brain's frontal lobe, which controls decision making. Laboratory mice that are isolated early in life have impaired cognitive abilities as they age. These experimental animals also have fewer brain cell branches, and the myelin insulation of their neuronal axons is thinner compared to mice that were not isolated.

It's not surprising that our brains have evolved to make us social beings. Our ancestors who were able to form and maintain relationships had the evolutionary advantage of becoming a group that could better defend against predators and search for food and shelter than an individual. Over hundreds of thousands of years, more socially adept people nurtured this survival advantage, which became programmed into their genes and hardwired into their brains.

The Social Brain
An entire investigative field known as *social neuroscience* has begun to unravel the complicated brain circuitry that controls our interactions with each other. This area of study is elucidating how and why we connect with other people through conversations, body language, and even touch.

Psychologist Dr. James Coan at the University of Virginia and his collaborators explored the brain effects of holding a spouse's hand. The investigators used MRI scanning to record brain responses to the stress of receiving a small electric shock. They found that the emotional support of holding a spouse's hand turned off the frontal lobe brain area that manages pain anticipation. The brain's hypothalamus, a deep brain area that controls stress hormone release, also showed less activity from hand holding. The researchers also found that holding hands had a greater antianxiety effect on volunteers from strong marriages. When the volunteers held the hand of a stranger, their brain's stress response was barely reduced at all. The findings suggest that holding hands with someone you love can have a profound effect on the deepest parts of your brain that controls stress.

Each person's ability to connect with friends and acquaintances varies, and some people are more challenged than others. At the extreme are those who suffer from autism, a disorder that involves difficulties in communicating and forming meaningful relationships. Patients with autism are reluctant to make eye contact and shy away from face-to-face conversations. Sustaining direct eye contact can convey intimacy as well as threats, and autistic individuals have trouble comprehending such nonverbal messages.

Scientists at the University of Wisconsin used MRI scans to study the brain structure of autistic traits. They focused on the relationship of maintaining eye contact and the size of the amygdala, a brain region that controls emotional responses. The investigators found that the volume of the amygdala was much smaller in autistic people than in people with normal social skills, and the autistic volunteers had substantial difficulties maintaining eye contact. The siblings of the autistic subjects also demonstrated a subtle reluctance to make eye contact, reflecting a genetic component to autistic traits.

Our minds draw us to others, and the rejection we feel if people snub us is sometimes comparable to physical pain. Research has pinpointed several brain regions that are highly sensitive to both the loss of a relationship and physical pain. University of Michigan investigators have shown that the same brain areas that activate when people feel rejected from an unwanted romantic breakup also respond to physical pain. Using MRI scanning, the investigators studied brain activity in 40 volunteers who had recently been rejected by a partner. The study subjects viewed photos of their previous partner and also were subjected to a mild physical pain. The somatosensory cortex, an area near the top of the head, and the insula, a frontal lobe region, were affected when experiencing either this emotional or physical pain.

Live Longer and Smarter with Friends

Social interactions cause our brains to release oxytocin, a hormone that fights against the negative effects of stress. Women, who tend to be more social than men, are more sensitive to the effects of oxytocin. This social, feel-good hormone reduces stress in people of every age.

Spending time with family and friends increases oxytocin levels and reduces stress. Having a chance to talk about our problems helps put our worries into perspective. These interactions reduce levels of cortisol and other stress hormones. Less stress and less cortisol can lower our risk for Alzheimer's, heart disease, and diabetes — all conditions that threaten our mind health.

When we are more connected to others, we feel better and actually live longer. Researchers at Harvard University found that spending time with family and friends increases the number of years we can expect to live. In their decade-long study of nearly 3,000 older adults, the investigators measured degrees of social engagement by recording the amount of time spent

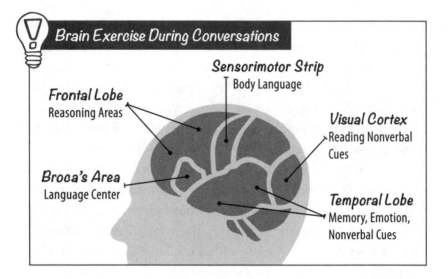

Brain Exercise During Conversations

Sensorimotor Strip
Body Language

Frontal Lobe
Reasoning Areas

Visual Cortex
Reading Nonverbal
Cues

Broca's Area
Language Center

Temporal Lobe
Memory, Emotion,
Nonverbal Cues

eating meals with others, playing team sports and games, and other social activities. They found that people engaged in more social interaction had a 20 percent greater likelihood of extended life expectancy.

When we spend time with other people, we have a greater sense of belonging and feel less alone. Friendly interactions elevate self-esteem and confidence. Having a chat with a friend provides a form of brain exercise as well. When thinking of what to say next or contemplating what someone just said, we're working out our neurons in many different brain regions. A brief, stimulating discussion will exercise neural circuits controlling language and reasoning, which are located in the brain's frontal lobe, as well as the medial temporal lobe memory centers. You'll respond to nonverbal cues to maintain eye contact and read body language, which triggers your temporal lobe and visual cortex, and your own nonverbal expressions will activate the sensorimotor strip at the top of your brain. If the discussion gets heated, you should expect your temporal lobe emotional center, the amygdala, to get involved as well.

Dr. Oscar Ybarra and associates studied what happens to our cognitive abilities as a result of a stimulating discussion. Compared to a control task of watching a sit-com rerun, a brief 10-minute conversation results in significant improvements in memory and speed of mental processing. Continuing such conversations over the years may be a key to protecting brain health since remaining social may slow age-related cognitive decline. Large-scale longitudinal studies suggest that avoiding loneliness may lower the risk for developing dementia by as much as 60 percent.

Connecting with the Right People

Ellen was already running late as she backed the car out of the garage. She wished she hadn't agreed to go to another one of Cindy and Ron's dinner parties. Cindy loved hosting these dinners and was the first to say that she "knew just about everybody." Ellen was almost sure they would seat her next to another single gentleman they'd invited who was supposed to charm her. Her friends meant well, but in the two years since her husband, Bruce, had died, they'd spent countless hours trying to distract her with lunches, shopping, parties, and other activities that Ellen was growing tired of.

When Ellen got to the party, everyone was already sitting down to dinner. Not surprisingly, she was seated between Cindy and a guy named Phillip, who immediately asked her what line of work she was in. Before Ellen could finish telling him about the gallery she used to curate, he jumped in, pontificating about all the artwork he had just purchased for his new beach house and how much he loved driving out there on weekends in his convertible Mercedes. He said she should come out with him one weekend and see his collection. Ellen made a mental note to never do that.

When she got home, Ellen felt a little down. It seemed like no matter how hard she tried, she just didn't feel connected with anyone in her life, not even Cindy and Ron. Luckily it was three hours earlier in California and she could still call Rose, her old college roommate and best buddy. Even though they hadn't seen each other in years, whenever they talked it was like no time had passed. The two convulsed in laughter when Ellen told Rose about Phillip's new beach house and his Mercedes convertible. Rose didn't know how Ellen had kept a straight face.

Talking to Rose always comforted Ellen. She didn't need to put on a happy face or avoid saying how much she missed Bruce. Before they got off the phone, Rose mentioned their upcoming fortieth college reunion and insisted that Ellen stay with her when she came to Los Angeles. Ellen said she wasn't planning to go to the reunion. She didn't want to show up without Bruce and spend the entire evening telling everyone what happened.

Rose wouldn't have it. She said Ellen couldn't just stop living now that Bruce was gone, and how many more reunions were they going to have? Besides, didn't Ellen want to see how fat and bald all their old boyfriends had become? Ellen wavered; it would be nice to spend some time with Rose, and getting out of town for a few days might be good for her.

When her taxi pulled up in front of Rose's house, Ellen got nervous. Would it be awkward staying with Rose after all these years? Should she have booked a hotel? Rose flung open the door and wrapped Ellen in a bear hug. They both started crying and Ellen's worries disappeared. They didn't stop talking and laughing until two in the morning, when they both crawled off to their bedrooms.

During the four days leading up to the reunion, Rose and Ellen had a fantastic time — it was like the old days when they would visit museums, see movies with subtitles, and dance to oldies in their pajamas. The reunion was fun, too.

On her flight home, Ellen settled in to watch the movie. As the ridiculous plot unfolded about a wealthy middle-aged man desperate to find a wife before he lost his inheritance, Ellen had an epiphany. Her loneliness since Bruce passed was not about her inability to connect with people; she just wasn't enjoying the people she had chosen to connect with. She'd been wasting time with things like Cindy's dinner parties and the superficial chatter about all the people Cindy knew and their material things. She yearned to have more friends like Rose in her life — friends with intellectual and cultural interests, who were fun to be around.

Back home, Ellen made a concerted effort to get involved with new activities. She contacted people she'd met through the gallery, started taking golf lessons, and volunteered as a docent at the modern art museum.

Good Versus Not-So-Good Friends

Many of us remain in friendships longer than we should. To get a sense of whether a particular friendship is one you want to nurture, ask yourself the following questions:

- Do you feel comfortable asking your friend for help when you need it?
  ☐ Yes ☐ No
- Does your friend offer and provide help when you ask for it?
  ☐ Yes ☐ No
- Do you have a lot in common with your friend?
  ☐ Yes ☐ No
- Does this person seldom gossip?
  ☐ Yes ☐ No
- Would you trust this friend with very personal information about yourself
  ☐ Yes ☐ No
- Do the two of you rarely get into arguments?
  ☐ Yes ☐ No
- Does your friend ever tell you sincerely that you are a good friend?
  ☐ Yes ☐ No
- Would you describe this person as a kind individual?
  ☐ Yes ☐ No
- Does your friend rarely do something mean to someone else or to you?
  ☐ Yes ☐ No

If you answered "no" to several of these questions, you might consider spending less time with this person and nurturing other relationships in your life.

The next time Cindy invited her to a dinner party, Ellen polite-ly declined. She was hosting her book club that evening. Cindy demanded to know whose book club it was. Ellen said, "Some-body I met at the museum — I'm sure you don't know her."

Sharing interests fosters our relationships, and for Ellen the lack of intellectual stimulation from the people she was spend-ing time with left her feeling isolated and alone. Social scien-tists have explained how we each have a tendency to create a close inner circle of friends. For most people, the size of that inner circle remains consistent over the years, even though the friends who comprise that circle may change. It's often help-ful to take periodic inventory of our inner circle of friends to make sure that we're spending our time with people we really care about.

Good Habits Are Contagious

Common denominators bring people together — we often meet potential friends at work, parties, or in the neighborhood. We tend to adopt traits of those closest to us by taking on similar habits and viewpoints. Of course, we seek out people with mu-tual interests and sensibilities, but to keep our brains healthy and young, it's a good idea to spend time with health-minded individuals; this increases the likelihood of our adopting and maintaining brain-healthy habits. Whether your best friend hangs out at the neighborhood fitness center or prefers drink-ing beer and watching sports will make a difference in how you spend your time.

Susan, a 56-year-old office manager, met Tom, a trial at-torney, at her tennis club. He was attractive and interesting — she loved hearing about his unusual cases. Tom was clearly the most intriguing man she had met since her divorce two years ago.

Susan loved playing sports. When they started dating, Tom joined her in tennis and jogging, her favorite pastimes, but after a while these outdoor activities gave way to late-night dinners and parties with his lawyer buddies.

Susan enjoyed being with Tom, but the more time they spent together, the less she played tennis or exercised. Their late-night dates were interfering with her sleep; she started gaining a little weight, and she was even late for work a few times.

As they finished supper one night at Tom's favorite Italian restaurant, he suggested they meet some of his friends at a nearby bar for a nightcap. Susan said she'd had enough to drink and she had to be at the office early in the morning. She suggested they meet for a run after work the next day. Tom got defensive — he didn't appreciate her suggestion that he drank too much, and he thought she liked his friends. Not wanting to get into an argument, Susan backed off and agreed to join Tom for the drink.

The next morning Susan woke up hungover and showed up late for work again. She realized that her relationship with Tom was not working and decided to give him an ultimatum: either they cool it on the partying, or they stop seeing each other. Tom got defensive again and said if she wanted to take a break, that was fine with him.

Susan felt hurt and missed Tom at first, but she stuck to her guns. She knew she couldn't continue the relationship the way it was going. It was bad for her health and her career.

After a couple weeks, Tom came around. He apologized and told her how much he missed her. He was ready to clean up his act and suggested they meet that weekend for a few sets of tennis. Susan agreed and offered to buy the drinks afterwards — at the juice bar.

Sometimes relationships that begin well eventually lead to negative and destructive behavior. Toxic relationships complicate people's lives and cause frustration, anger, and guilt. Remaining in one or more toxic friendships leads to stressful relationship clutter.

Fine-Tune Your Listening Skills

One reason that people often do not connect to one another is that they don't focus their attention during conversations. Here is an exercise that can strengthen your ability to avoid distractions and heighten your listening skills. It's best to attempt this exercise with a close friend or partner. It doesn't take much time but can really enhance your attention and let the other person know you care about what they're saying.

Ask your partner to discuss an issue that has personal meaning — perhaps a recent problem, a long-term challenge, or an upcoming event. Tell your partner to focus on feelings and avoid criticism, and you should do the same when it's your turn to talk. Avoiding personal attacks will reduce defensiveness and help the listener to focus more on understanding. Set your timer for two minutes while your partner talks.

As you listen, maintain eye contact and try not to interrupt — this will help you to pay attention. Your mind may wander or you may have an emotional reaction to the conversation, but try to ignore those distractions and bring your focus back to listening.

After your two minutes of listening, reset your timer for two minutes and switch roles so that you are the speaker and your partner is the listener. You may wish to continue discussing the same topic or pick an entirely different one. While speaking, continue to avoid criticism and focus on expressing your feelings.

The last step is to discuss how each of you felt about the exercise. Did it make you feel closer? Was it frustrating? Was it exhilarating?

We often continue unhealthy interactions simply out of habit. It can be uncomfortable to cut off someone whom you've known for many years, and the negativity you get from that person can become so chronic that you don't even realize it's there. Recognizing unhealthy friendships and attempting to clear out relationship clutter reduces stress and leaves more time to spend in healthy relationships.

It is possible to repair a relationship that is not entirely toxic but has simply deteriorated over the years. It might involve someone who used to have a positive influence in your life and you feel it's worth the effort required to mend the friendship. If you choose to work on a relationship, it's helpful to carve out dedicated time to get together, attempt to share your true feelings, and see if you can resolve your differences or conflicts.

The Empathic Brain

Hundreds of thousands of years of evolution have created an intricate and complex neural system in our brains that helps us to understand one another. The ability to imagine and comprehend what someone else is feeling — what we call *empathy* — is a powerful mental force that serves to connect human beings, and those social connections help maintain brain health.

We are all born with the capacity to empathize, but fine-tuning those abilities involves practice and maturity. Research has shown that experiencing empathy is more of a challenge when we are young. Scientists at San Diego State University studied empathic abilities in teenagers by asking them to observe facial expressions depicting various emotional states. Compared to other age groups, the 11- and 12-year-olds took the greatest amount of time to identify the emotions of the faces presented to them.

Other research by Dr. Sarah-Jayne Blakemore and colleagues at University College in London has confirmed that, like a fine wine, empathy gets better with age. They also pinpointed some of the brain regions involved in empathic responses. The scientists performed MRI scans on adolescents aged 11 to 17 and compared the results to those of young adults aged 21 to 37 years. During the brain scans, the volunteers were asked to make everyday decisions, like when to eat dinner, when to get up in the morning, and when to go to school or work. The two groups used different brain regions to make these decisions: the adolescents tapped their temporal lobes (underneath the temples) while the young adults utilized an area in their prefrontal cortex that monitors decisions that affect other people. The investigators also tested how quickly the volunteers could determine the impact of their decisions on someone else's well-being. The older volunteers answered these questions at a much quicker pace thanks to their more developed frontal lobe decision-making abilities.

UCLA investigators at the Ahmanson-Lovelace Brain Mapping Center performed MRI scans to pinpoint the empathy center of the brain. They scanned volunteers while they studied photos of faces expressing happiness, sadness, surprise, and other emotions, and while they attempted to mirror those facial expression. The scientists found that both observing the expressions and imitating them lit up the same brain region — the

---

How Empathic Are You?

Some people are born more empathic than others. They're better at understanding someone else's feelings and perspective and are more effective at conveying their understanding. Answer the following questions to get an idea of your current empathic abilities.

- Do you sometimes get bored when people talk about their feelings?
  ☐ Yes   ☐ No

- Is it difficult to place another person's interests ahead of your own?
  ☐ Yes   ☐ No

- Do you prefer distancing yourself from friends who upset you rather then discussing your differences?
  ☐ Yes   ☐ No

- Are you uncomfortable talking about your feelings?
  ☐ Yes   ☐ No

- Do you tend to change topics in a conversation when it gets too personal?
  ☐ Yes   ☐ No

- When you are upset, do you prefer to be alone rather than discuss it with a friend?
  ☐ Yes   ☐ No

If you answered yes to one or more of the questions, then focusing on developing better empathy skills might improve your social connections and brain health. Even if you scored well on this brief quiz, building empathy skills can still enhance your relationships and be worth the effort.

insula. This oval-shaped area at the juncture separating the temporal and frontal lobes translates our experiences with the outside world into internal feelings. The activity in the insula was greater during the imitation phase of the experiment than the observation phase.

To get a better sense of the power of empathy, Dr. Tania Singer's group at the Institute of Neurology at University College in London studied couples in love. They mapped the brain activity of one partner while receiving a small electric shock, and also while watching his or her mate appear to experience the same pain. The researchers found that both the insula and the anterior cingulate (in the frontal lobe) were activated — whether the subject actually experienced the pain or simply believed their partner was experiencing it.

Growing up with empathic role models is an effective way to develop empathy. Over the years we also experience our own feelings of happiness and suffering that make it easier for us to understand others when they have similar experiences. In addition to the emotional wisdom we gain as we age, we can increase our empathy by mastering these two basic skills:

- *Attentive listening.* It's often said that the best conversationalists are those who know how to listen. Focusing attention and setting aside distractions, such as phones and other gadgets, is critical. Try not to interrupt the speaker to express your own feelings and reactions.

- *Expressing understanding.* The real power of empathy emerges when you communicate your understanding back to someone after they have expressed their feelings. This can be done by restating what you perceive as the other person's perspective. You might use simple statements like, "Let me see if I have this right . . ." You can also ask follow-up questions to get additional detail, which shows both your interest and acceptance.

Brief Empathy Exercise

Your friend tells you about the following upsetting situation:

"My husband is really getting to me. I can barely look him in the eye I'm so angry. I can't stand that he spends more time with his golf buddies than with me, and he forgot to get me a present on my birthday. I really do love him, but we don't have any romance in our lives."

Before proceeding, spend a moment considering how you might respond.

Here are several possibilities:

Offer unsolicited advice. "You're crazy to criticize him. I know he loves you, and no relationship is perfect." This kind of unsolicited advice is usually unwelcome. If you lecture your friend, she probably won't feel supported. The desire to fix somebody else's problem often stems from our own anxiety that the conflict is causing us.

Share your own experience. "I know exactly what you're feeling. My ex-husband was really a jerk — his job was always more important than our marriage." You may be trying to help by relating your similar experience, but the timing could be wrong. Instead of showing empathy, you are switching the focus to your own problems and suggesting that your marital solution could be right for your friend.

Reflect and mirror. "I didn't know you felt that way. I can see that you are upset and angry. Tell me more about what's going on." This response is much more empathic. Repeating back how your friend feels indicates that you are listening, and it shows your interest and concern.

Humor Brings People Together

A good laugh not only releases tension, it can improve our health and help us feel more connected to others. Norman Cousins described how watching the Marx Brothers and other comedians helped him battle ankylosing spondylitis, a painful and crippling arthritic disease. Social scientists are revealing how humor can bring people together and help solve their relationship disputes.

Psychologist Dr. Alice Isen and colleagues have found that watching a brief comedy film of TV bloopers facilitates creative solutions to problems. When we get someone else's joke, we share an understanding of life, relationships, or whatever topic

Knowing When to Joke

Although humor can bring people together and cut tension in a relationship, there is a time and place for everything, especially jokes. To determine whether going for a laugh may help or hurt your conversation, ask yourself some of the following questions:

- Are you and your friend conveying nonverbal signals of warmth or hostility?
- Does your friend have a sense of humor that clicks with yours?
- Are you calm enough to make your joke work?
- Are you trying to communicate positive feelings, or is your joke an attempt to express anger or resentment?
- Is your joke at someone else's expense and might your friend take offense?

the joke addresses. When we laugh at the same thing as others, we let them know that we see the situation in a similar way. In this way, humor can communicate a mutual perspective that can help people deal with uncomfortable topics.

Joking around can bolster brain health through the mental calisthenics of juxtaposing information in new and funny ways. Studies of how the brain processes humor indicate that a complex network of neurons communicate when we laugh. Laughter triggers the brain's dopamine reward systems, as well as left brain networks that help us resolve any logical incongruities a joke may present.

Humor also helps our brains stay young by lowering stress levels. Watching a half-hour television comedy has been shown to lower blood biomarkers of stress. Laughing also blunts hunger stimuli and helps people control emotional eating, which can lead to weight gain.

Sex, Love, and Brain Health

Sex can heighten intimacy and help keep our brains young. Animal studies indicate that sexual activity lowers stress levels and stimulates cell growth in the hippocampal memory center. Dr.

Benedetta Leuner and associates at Princeton University and Claremont Colleges exposed adult male rats to a sexually receptive female once daily for 14 consecutive days and measured cell growth in the hippocampus. Immediately following sexual activity, neuron growth in the hippocampus increased. After two weeks, the scientists counted even more neurons, which had sprouted new branches for cellular communication.

A healthy sex life not only makes us feel good, it may contribute to longer life expectancy. In a 10-year longitudinal study, Professor George Davey Smith of the University of Bristol in England found a 50 percent lower mortality rate in men who had more frequent orgasms. Sexual excitement and orgasm releases the hormone DHEA, which naturally declines in the body after age 30. DHEA has been found to protect heart health, which may explain why greater sexual activity may extend life expectancy. Endorphins and other hormones released during sex and orgasm also lead to a relaxation response and better sleep, which further promote brain health.

Our body's ability to fight off infection also improves when we are sexually active. Immunoglobulin A is an antibody that protects us from infectious diseases, and one study found that college students who had sex once or twice a week had a 30 percent higher immunoglobulin A level compared to students who were sexually abstinent.

If your level of sexual activity is not what it used to be, no worries — several studies indicate that physical expressions of love without intercourse can bolster brain and body health. Just hugging someone can lower blood pressure. Research has shown that couples react better to stress after holding hands and hugging. Other studies indicate that men who feel loved and supported by their spouses have a lower rate of developing angina, the chest pain caused by an inadequate blood supply to the heart.

The hormone and neurotransmitter oxytocin, sometimes referred to as the love molecule, works to strengthen relationships, trust, and our feelings of attachment to one another. Our brains release oxytocin when we hold hands, kiss, and cuddle, and when we are sexually aroused, blood levels of oxytocin rise significantly. Along with dopamine and norepinephrine, oxytocin plays a large role in pair bonding. It also helps lower levels of fear, pain, and stress.

New Technology Helps Keep Our Friends Close

During the last two decades, we've experienced an extraordinary influx of new technologies that help us stay in touch with friends, family, and associates. Desktops, smartphones, tablets, and other gadgets have become essential tools that enhance our work efficiency and social lives.

Not long ago, if you wanted to connect quickly with someone in your office, you'd probably call her on a regular phone. She would either answer, the line would be busy, or she wasn't there. Today, you might first call her landline, leave a voice mail, and then try her cell phone and leave a second message. You could also text, e-mail, instant message, or connect with her through Facebook. But if all else fails, you can resort to old-school methods and walk across the hall to her office.

Our brains enjoy the novelty of new technology, but all the pings and buzzes tend to distract us from our work, as well as our face-to-face interactions. We can take steps to keep our tech lives from interfering with our off-line lives by silencing or turning off our devices in social situations.

Although our smartphones and computers now make it possible to instantly converse with people throughout the world, we need to remain mindful of what we communicate with each of these methods. Everything we text or post on the Internet can become public information and is open to various interpretations or misinterpretations. A long series of e-mails is not always the most efficient way to address a complex interpersonal issue. Most of us would agree that ending a romantic

---

Healthy Relationships for Better Brain Health

- Remain involved with friends and family because social bonds strengthen brain cell connections.
- Conversations are mental calisthenics that bolster neural networks. Engage in daily discussions about topics of interest to keep your neural circuits agile.
- Spending time with health-conscious people promotes your own brain and body health because good habits are contagious.
- Try to let go of toxic relationships so you have more time to spend with people you truly like.
- Practice paying full attention when you listen to others. Try not to interrupt or misinterpret their feelings.
- Empathy is a powerful social skill that can be learned and developed. Try to share your feelings without criticizing, and let your friends know you understand how they feel.
- Use humor to help diffuse tension and become closer to others, but make sure the timing and situation is right. Avoid negative jokes that express anger or resentment.

---

relationship through a text message or Facebook post may not be the best approach. And although videoconferencing is a pretty close two-dimensional version of a human interaction, it does not seem to have the same impact as an in-person encounter.

Face-to-face conversations are still the best way to convey emotions, empathy, and nonverbal cues. But in our busy modern world, they are not always possible. With the advent of more powerful Wi-Fi and broadband connections, as well as new technologies in development, including three-dimensional imaging and virtual reality techniques, I have no doubt that Internet conversations will continue to become even more compelling and realistic in the future.

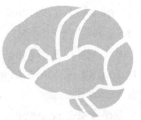

CHAPTER EIGHT

Mind Your Medicine

"Be careful about reading health books. You may die of a misprint."

—*Mark Twain*

I HAVE ATTENDED MANY SCIENTIFIC meetings on memory and aging, where I've met investigators from around the world with varying expertise and points of view. Our discussions sometimes led to new collaborations and studies that resulted in novel scientific advances.

At one of these workshops, there was a heated debate about the mild memory slips that affect nearly everyone by the time they reach age 45. Most of the attendees were doctors from research institutes and universities, but a few people were from the pharmaceutical industry and there was one official from the Food and Drug Administration (FDA). I liked that we had someone from the FDA because that's the agency that decides whether a new drug meets the standards for approval.

Someone asked whether the FDA would ever approve a medicine for treating mild age-associated memory complaints, such as a drug to help us remember someone's name or where we put our keys. Everyone was skeptical that such a "smart drug" could get approved. The lone FDA official felt differently — just because a drug isn't targeting Alzheimer's or some other brain disease, he said, didn't mean that it couldn't be approved for an age-related condition. Don't many people wear glasses or contact lenses or undergo LASIK surgery to improve normal decline in vision? This age-related condition is not a disease, but we still have treatments for it.

The Placebo Effect

Whether a medicine is effective or not depends on its ability to work better than an inactive placebo pill, and the FDA has specific regulatory requirements for drugs or devices to pass this test. For medicines to be approved, both their safety and effectiveness must be confirmed in double-blind, placebo-controlled clinical trials, which means that neither the doctors conducting the study nor the patients enrolled know who is taking the real medicine and who is taking an inactive placebo.

Placebos can actually make us feel better, at least temporarily, and most doctors have observed this effect. A survey of physicians in academic medical centers revealed that nearly half of the respondents use placebos in their clinical practice, and 96 percent believed that placebos do have therapeutic effects. Some experts estimate that we can observe a temporary placebo effect about 30 percent of the time.

The physiological effects of placebos can be observed in brain scans. Dr. Tor Wager and colleagues at the University of Michigan used MRI scans to show that when volunteers anticipating pain took a placebo painkiller that they believed was real, they had decreased brain activity in areas controlling pain sensation.

But this real placebo effect wears off after a while. In the first clinical trial of a drug developed for the treatment of Alzheimer's dementia, the drug and placebo effects were the same for

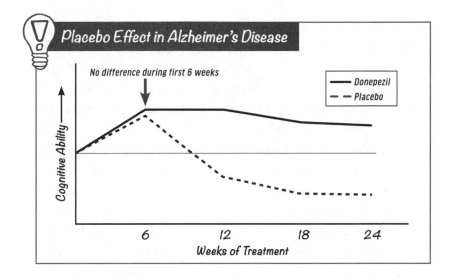

Placebo Effect in Alzheimer's Disease

No difference during first 6 weeks

— Donepezil
– – Placebo

Cognitive Ability

6   12   18   24

Weeks of Treatment

the first six weeks of the study. After that, the patients receiving the placebo got worse and those taking the real drug did better (see figure).

There are several possible explanations for why the placebo worked during those first six weeks of the study. It may have been the expectations of the caregivers and patients that this new medicine really did something, or perhaps the nice nurses and doctors who spent time with the patients made them feel better. Had the study ended after six weeks, the investigators would have incorrectly concluded that the medicine didn't work any better than the placebo.

Partnering with Your Doctor

Even though age increases the risk for chronic medical conditions and dementia, today's older adults are enjoying longer, healthier, and more active lives thanks to modern healthcare and medicines. Taking care of our health is essential for keeping our brains young, and establishing a good relationship with a trusted physician is important.

Traditionally, doctors took a paternalistic attitude toward their patients: the physician acted like a parent, telling the patient what to do, and the patient followed the doctor's orders — and we still call them orders. Today, this paternalistic healthcare model has been abandoned for one that emphasizes patient autonomy and shared decision making with the doctor. Patients are becoming knowledgeable healthcare consumers, and their values and perspectives are now included in the doctor's evaluation and treatment planning.

Patients have also become savvier healthcare consumers thanks to the Internet and other media, which provide the latest information on medical research, drugs, and supplements. Patients often hear about apparent breakthroughs even before their doctors read about them in their medical journals. In 2014, the Pew Research Internet Project reported that 87 percent of US adults used the Internet and 72 percent of those Internet users said they searched online for health information within the past year. More than half of the Internet searchers who self-diagnosed sought help from their doctors. The challenge is finding valid information on the web, and your doctor can help you make sense of what you've read and help you to discern between what is real and what may be hype.

It's a good idea to discuss the potential benefits and risks of any diagnostic or treatment option with your doctor so you share in the decision making. Some people, however, still hold on to older paternalistic values. A patient may be reluctant to speak candidly with her doctor, who may seem critical of her lifestyle habits. She may think that her doctor would be insulted if he knew she had sought a second opinion. Another patient may feel he will disappoint his doctor if he has not taken the prescribed medicines. Because your physical health has such important implications for your mind health, it's best to overcome such fears and strive to partner with your physician.

Preparing for your appointments will help you to make the most of the relatively brief amount of time available for most doctor visits. To ensure that your questions are answered, write them down in advance and bring the list to your appointment. Also, if you are

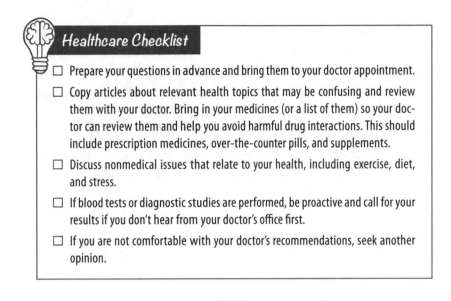

Healthcare Checklist

☐ Prepare your questions in advance and bring them to your doctor appointment.

☐ Copy articles about relevant health topics that may be confusing and review them with your doctor. Bring in your medicines (or a list of them) so your doctor can review them and help you avoid harmful drug interactions. This should include prescription medicines, over-the-counter pills, and supplements.

☐ Discuss nonmedical issues that relate to your health, including exercise, diet, and stress.

☐ If blood tests or diagnostic studies are performed, be proactive and call for your results if you don't hear from your doctor's office first.

☐ If you are not comfortable with your doctor's recommendations, seek another opinion.

confused about a magazine or web article, bring in a copy so you and your doctor can review it together. Your physician may also ask you to bring in all your medicines to check for possible harmful drug interactions. Be sure to bring up any issues about diet, exercise, stress, or mental symptoms you may be experiencing.

Treating Physical Illnesses Can Save Your Brain

Physical illnesses such as pneumonia, flu, anemia, thyroid imbalance, or even a urinary tract infection can lead to temporary confusion or memory loss. When I evaluate patients with memory issues, I always look for any medical conditions that can affect brain function. Although most medical causes can be identified after a physical exam and lab tests, sometimes patients don't follow up on their doctor's treatment recommendations.

Charlie was one of those patients. He was looking forward to his 70th birthday and proud of the fact that he was in great shape, had a full head of hair, and still enjoyed a fairly regular sex life with his wife, Angela. He almost never got sick and only took a couple of Tylenols once in a while if he was sore from working out. He loved it when people were surprised at his age.

Of course, Charlie worked hard to stay toned and keep the weight off his belly. He had always been athletic — in high school, he ran track and was captain of the tennis team. He still played tennis twice a week, jogged almost every morning, and swam laps at the gym.

After his yearly physical, Charlie waited in his doctor's office to hear the results of his electrocardiogram and other tests. The doctor came in and greeted him.

"What's the good news, Doc?"

"Everything looks fine, Charlie, but you told the nurse you weren't taking your statin meds for your cholesterol."

"You know I hate taking pills. Besides, I've really cut back on meat and eggs. I feel great."

"A year ago your cholesterol level was 220. If today's test comes in over 200, I want you to take the medicine."

"How about I cut out all red meat, eggs, and dairy? And I can exercise more."

"Those are good ideas, Charlie, but after age 60 the risk for heart disease and stroke go up anyway. I don't want you compounding that risk with high cholesterol."

"Fine, Doc, whatever you say."

Out to dinner Saturday night, Charlie ordered the salmon but reached for the butter for his bread. Angela looked surprised.

"Are you supposed to eat butter?"

"I can't cut out everything. I have to live."

"That's the point, Charlie. Don't play around with your cholesterol. It's not a joke."

"Do I look like I'm laughing? I'm almost a vegetarian and I've been swimming 10 extra laps all week — I practically live at the gym."

Angela sighed and moved the butter to the next table.

The next day they were playing doubles with their friends at the tennis club. Charlie moved into position to return a serve, but he didn't swing as the ball passed by him. He dropped his racquet and looked at it, confused.

"Are you okay, honey?" Angela asked.

"I don't know, my right hand feels . . ."

"What? What does it feel?"

"It feels . . . I can't feel it . . ."

Charlie was silent — he couldn't speak. They helped him sit down on a bench and called 911.

Angela sat nervously next to Charlie's bed in the emergency room. The feeling in his hand was back and he was talking normally. A young doctor came in and said that Charlie's brain scan ruled out a stroke. He'd had a TIA, or transient ischemic attack. The doctor explained that it was like a mini-stroke, but the symptoms were temporary and there was no permanent damage.

Angela hugged Charlie, relieved. The doctor told them that a TIA should be taken as a wake-up call. It was both a warning that Charlie could have a stroke later and an opportunity to begin doing things to avoid it. He said Charlie's vitals were fine and wondered if he had high cholesterol. Angela shot Charlie an "I told you so" look. Charlie told the doctor that he had a prescription for statin drugs at home and he would start taking them right away.

Charlie followed up with his own physician every other week for the next two months. His medication, low-cholesterol diet, and extra exercise helped bring his cholesterol level down to 190, and he vowed to do everything to keep it there.

Charlie didn't realize how much cholesterol levels could affect not only his physical health, but his cognitive abilities too. High cholesterol can cause plaque buildup in the arteries that can block normal blood flow to the brain and cause a stroke. It can also increase the risk for heart disease and atherosclerosis, which are both risk factors for stroke.

Left untreated, high cholesterol, hypertension, heart disease, diabetes, and other age-related medical illnesses can threaten brain health through cerebrovascular damage or injury to the brain's supporting blood vessels, leading to TIAs or strokes.

Do Cholesterol Drugs Help Memory?

In general, taking a statin cholesterol-lowering drug is good for the brain. A number of investigations including thousands of volunteers age 75 and older indicate that taking statins does bolster brain health and lower the risk for Alzheimer's disease. However, if someone already has Alzheimer's dementia, treatment with a statin drug has no better effect than taking a placebo. In a small number of people, statin medicines can cause memory loss or confusion as a side effect. Fortunately, when these patients stop taking the medicine, their memory improves.

Fortunately for Charlie, his symptoms were only temporary and he began taking medication immediately.

Cholesterol-Lowering Statins

High blood levels of cholesterol, particularly the harmful LDL form, contribute to the accumulation of fatty plaques in arteries throughout the body that put the brain at risk for strokes. Exercise, diet, and statin drugs can control blood cholesterol levels and lower a person's future risk for strokes, dementia, and Alzheimer's disease.

Statins may protect our brains by blocking the liver's production of an enzyme necessary for cholesterol synthesis. These drugs also have anti-inflammatory effects and raise levels of nitric oxide, which helps keep blood vessel walls flexible enough for ample blood flow. Research also has linked cholesterol to the amyloid plaques deposited in the brains of Alzheimer's victims, suggesting that statins might protect brain health by disrupting amyloid brain deposition.

Drugs for Hypertension

By age 65, approximately half the population has high blood pressure, and untreated hypertension can increase the risk for cognitive decline. Chronic hypertension may impair memory because it thickens and stiffens blood vessels in the brain. Under high pressure, these stiffened blood vessels can rupture and leak blood into brain tissue. This process can eventually cause a stroke, which is defined as brain cell death that results in loss of physical or mental function, or both.

Although antihypertensive medicines can treat high blood pressure, the medicine is more effective when patients also engage in healthy lifestyles. Regular exercise, a low-salt diet, quitting smoking, and limiting excessive alcohol and food consumption all help to control blood pressure. Our UCLA functional MRI studies show that the subtle brain injuries associated with high blood pressure may force our brains to work harder in order to remember things.

Anti-Inflammatory Drugs

During the past two decades, epidemiological studies have shown that people who take anti-inflammatory drugs lower their risk for Alzheimer's disease by as much as 60 percent after two years of use. These drugs, including ibuprofen (Motrin, Advil) and naproxen (Aleve), are usually used to treat the pain and inflammation from injuries and arthritis.

Anti-inflammatory medicines may protect the brain by fighting inflammatory responses to injury or infection. Numerous investigations suggest that Alzheimer's disease and other forms of neurodegeneration result from an inflamed brain. When pathologists examine the Alzheimer brain plaques under the microscope, they see inflammatory cells and debris surrounding the plaques. One theory holds that an inflammatory attack to rid the brain of amyloid protein could lead to cell death and memory loss, and anti-inflammatory drugs may block this damaging process. Other studies show that some anti-inflammatory drugs bind to amyloid plaques and may block their accumulation in the brain.

Anti-inflammatory drugs are not currently recommended as a brain protection treatment for several reasons. Even though the drugs may protect brain health in people with mild memory symptoms, they appear to accelerate cognitive decline in patients who have Alzheimer's dementia, and the tipping point when the drugs transition from helpful to harmful is not known. Anti-inflammatory drugs also have many side effects. In some people, the medicines can increase blood pressure, cause kidney problems, or lead to bleeding in the stomach. However, if your doctor is prescribing one of these drugs to help with your arthritis or another physical condition, it may also be protecting your brain. Scientists are still studying the effect of these medicines on brain health while they continue to research safer anti-inflammatory treatments.

Too Many Medicines

When I started focusing my work on geriatrics, I was taught to ask patients to bring all their medicines with them to their first

---

Tylenol Vs. Motrin

Most of us are aware of some of the differences between Tylenol and Motrin, but not everyone knows about the potential side effects of these common over-the-counter medicines. Tylenol (acetaminophen) is effective in treating pain and fever but has no impact on inflammation. If you sprain your ankle, Tylenol will reduce the pain you feel but do nothing to decrease swelling and redness, which are signs of the inflammatory response that repairs your damaged ankle.

Motrin/Advil (ibuprofen), Aleve (naproxen), and similar medicines are known as nonsteroidal anti-inflammatory drugs (or NSAIDs as doctors like to call them). These drugs will relieve pain and lower fever and also reduce inflammation. That can be particularly helpful for joint pain, swelling, and injuries. What limits more widespread use of NSAIDs is their potentially serious side effects, such as stomach bleeding, allergic reactions, and kidney and heart problems. It's always a good idea to take NSAIDs with food to minimize stomach irritation.

Because Tylenol doesn't cause side effects in most people, it is often assumed that it is completely safe. However, too much Tylenol can cause serious and life-threatening liver damage, so it's critically important, as with all medicines, to follow the recommended dosages. Combining alcohol and acetaminophen increases the risk of liver and kidney problems.

visit so I could see if any were helping or worsening their mental symptoms. Many of my patients showed up at the clinic with shopping bags full of medications, some of which had expired years earlier.

As we get older, chronic medical conditions can lead to the use of multiple prescription medicines with various side effects. Also, many over-the-counter drugs that people take without their doctor's supervision can have side effects. Sometimes combining prescription and over-the-counter medicines can cause potentially dangerous side effects.

I often consult with patients who have been seeing several different doctors who are prescribing various medications and no one is coordinating the treatment. Also, patients often change doctors over the years and may continue taking old prescriptions without the new doctor's awareness.

As we age, our bodies become more sensitive to drugs, and this is one reason that physical illnesses can make us more susceptible to adverse drug effects. The kidney and liver metabolize and excrete medicines, and these organs can become less efficient so the same dose of a medicine that a younger person takes may be too much for an older person. Older bodies also tend to have a greater proportion of fat, and drugs that dissolve in fat may become trapped in the body, leading to elevated toxic levels over time.

Anyone considering an over-the-counter medicine should check with their doctor or pharmacist about the indications and potential side effects. A lot of people don't realize that many over-the-counter antihistamines and sleeping medicines can cause memory loss. It turns out that these drugs contain chemicals that interfere with neurotransmitters in the brain that are necessary for memory function.

Too much of any medicine can cause side effects, especially in people who are particularly sensitive to drugs. Low or high thyroid levels can impair memory, but so can too much thyroid

> ### Valium-Induced Dementia
>
> Many patients take medicines to help with insomnia, but such sedatives can lead to confusion or memory loss during the day. Early in my training as a geriatric psychiatrist, I treated a patient whose initial diagnosis was Alzheimer's disease. For several years, he had gotten into the habit of taking 10 milligrams of Valium (diazepam) every night for sleep, as well as another anxiety medicine during the day. I suspected that these drugs might be contributing to his memory symptoms, so I gradually discontinued them. He initially had trouble sleeping and felt more anxiety during the day but was thrilled when his memory loss cleared up. He had been misdiagnosed with Alzheimer's disease — he did not have a permanent dementia but a reversible one resulting from medication side effects and interactions.
>
> Although Valium and other anti-anxiety drugs do calm people down and help them with insomnia, these medicines can accumulate in the body and impair memory — especially in older individuals. If such drugs are necessary, I prefer prescribing newer ones that do not remain in the body as long and are less likely to cause side effects.

medication. Prednisone, bladder-control drugs, some antidepressants, and pain medicines can cause confusion and alter mood, so make sure you tell your doctor about what you're taking and any side effects you may experience.

Medicines to Treat Cognitive Impairment

Just over two decades ago, doctors had no treatments for the millions of patients suffering from Alzheimer's disease. Although a cure has yet to be discovered, several medicines are now available that treat the memory and other cognitive symptoms of the disease. Because Alzheimer's brains have a deficit of the neurotransmitter acetylcholine, most symptomatic medicines such as Aricept (donepezil), Exelon (rivastigmine), and Razadyne (galantamine) increase brain levels of acetylcholine. Adding on Namenda (memantine), which affects a different neurotransmitter, provides further cognitive benefits.

These medications have been approved for the treatment of Alzheimer's disease, but they also help patients with related illnesses, such as vascular dementia and dementia with Lewy bodies. The drugs not only temporarily benefit memory and thinking, but they can also lower levels of agitation and improve symptoms of depression. Side effects may include appetite decline, indigestion, nausea, slowed heart rate, and insomnia, but increasing the dosage gradually can help minimize such effects. One of the medicines, rivastigmine, comes in a transdermal patch form that has fewer digestive system side effects.

Some people with normal age-related memory complaints or mild cognitive impairment have undergone PET scans to determine if their brains show evidence of Alzheimer's disease. When someone's brain scan does show evidence of amyloid plaque or tangle buildup, they may be eager to take an anti-Alzheimer's medicine before their symptoms progress.

The following FDDNP-PET scans show how Alzheimer's plaques and tangles (white areas) are minimal in someone without memory symptoms (scan on left) but easily observed in someone who has MCI, or mild cognitive impairment (scan on right). A person's brain scan may show evidence of plaques and tangles even if their symptoms are very mild, but it's not yet

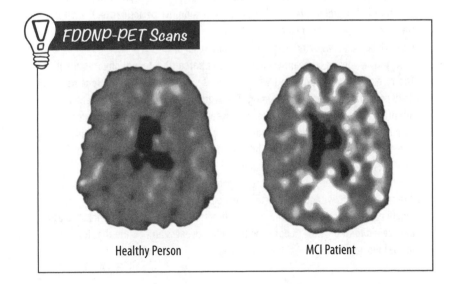

FDDNP-PET Scans

Healthy Person   MCI Patient clear if taking anti-dementia medicine will help prevent further cognitive decline, and for how long.

Our UCLA research group found that after 18 months of treatment, Aricept worked no better than a placebo in people with only mild age-associated memory complaints. Dr. Ron Petersen's study of patients who already had mild cognitive impairment showed that those taking Aricept were less likely to advance to Alzheimer's dementia after a year compared with those taking a placebo, but after three years there was no advantage.

Even though an antidepressant drug can cause memory side effects on occasion, many depressed patients experience improved memory abilities when their mood is elevated with treatment. As people age, mood and memory symptoms tend to occur together. Patients can get frustrated and depressed due to their awareness of memory loss. Lifting their mood

Can a Medical Device Boost Brainpower?

Wearing a headband may help keep your hair out of your eyes, but some people are wearing a new kind of headband that is more than just a fashion statement. It delivers a low dose of electricity to the brain in order to improve mood, raise pain thresholds, promote restful sleep, or bolster cognitive performance. Known as transcranial direct current stimulation, or tDCS, the technology has been tested in research labs and has demonstrated promising results.

A study involving 60 healthy volunteers compared tDCS to a phony treatment. The researchers were exploring whether the device augmented the benefits of daily computerized cognitive training. The study showed that tDCS did enhance attention and memory abilities after four weeks of follow-up. Other research has demonstrated improvements in reading efficiency and name recall, as well as benefits for patients with depression and neurological diseases — tDCS reduced the time they needed to master a particular skill.

Experts are concerned, however, that people may purchase these devices online and use them without adequate supervision. If electric current improves brain function in specific regions, it may worsen function in other areas. Further studies are needed to clarify how to optimize tDCS effectiveness and ensure that it is safe to use long-term.

can improve concentration and memory. Other times, symptoms of depression may reflect an underlying brain problem. The first generation of antidepressants, like amitriptyline (Elavil) or imipramine (Tofranil) worsened memory loss. Newer antidepressants, such as the SSRIs or selective serotonin reuptake inhibitors (e.g., Zoloft or Prozac), have fewer memory side effects.

Hormones for a Better Brain

Hormones are natural or synthetic chemicals that regulate body functions and can be used to treat many medical conditions. Patients with diabetes take the hormone insulin to ensure that their blood sugar levels are stable, and taking estrogen can reduce a woman's menopausal symptoms. Investigators have explored how hormones might enhance brain health and memory function. Although there is limited evidence of their effectiveness in boosting cognitive performance, muscle mass, and libido, many people still use them as supplements. They tout the fact that hormones are natural, but many don't realize that natural doesn't guarantee safety.

DHEA

Dehydroepiandrosterone (DHEA), a building block for the sex hormones estrogen and testosterone, may enhance libido, build muscle, and lower body weight. Some athletes take DHEA to improve strength, energy, and muscle mass, but the National Collegiate Athletic Association (NCAA) and National Football League (NFL) have banned its use.

The hormone has been shown to improve memory in laboratory animals, and some studies in human volunteers suggest that DHEA may benefit mood and memory. Large-scale human studies are not available to confirm whether its potential brain health benefits outweigh its risks. Side effects include increased cancer risk, facial hair growth, scalp balding, and acne.

HUMAN GROWTH HORMONE

Children with human growth hormone (HGH) deficiency can reach normal heights during adolescence thanks to replacement therapy. Because the body's levels of HGH decline with age, some people have used it to fight the physical and mental effects of aging. Potential hazards include pain, edema (swelling from increased fluid in the body's tissues), elevated cholesterol levels, growth of cancer cells, and increased risk of diabetes.

Investigators recently studied the effects of somatoliberin (a hormone that stimulates HGH release) on cognitive function in healthy older adults and patients with mild cognitive impairment. They injected either the hormone or a placebo under the skin of volunteers each evening for 20 weeks and found that those receiving the hormone had improved cognitive abilities. The scientists recommended longer-duration studies to further determine its therapeutic potential on brain health.

ESTROGEN

Estrogen declines at menopause, increasing a woman's risk of Alzheimer's dementia, and epidemiological studies indicate that estrogen replacement therapy lowers that risk. Such associations do not prove that estrogen has a direct brain effect, and placebo-controlled, double-blind trials of the cognitive effects of estrogen have yielded mixed results. Estrogen's potential to increase the risk of cancer, stroke, and heart disease make doctors cautious about prescribing it.

The Women's Health Initiative indicated that women aged 65 years or older who took the estrogen brand Premarin had a greater risk of dementia. However, other studies show that women taking hormone therapy earlier in life — around the time of menopause — have a lower dementia risk, suggesting that there may be a window of opportunity when estrogen can do more good for cognition than harm. Other research suggests that progestogen (another hormone often combined with estrogen replacement) may be more important in determining memory effects than the type of estrogen.

TESTOSTERONE

Testosterone gradually declines in men as they age, and about one out of five men 65 and older have abnormally low testosterone levels. Some men who have not been tested for low

Beware of Testosterone Supplements

Phil dreaded turning 60 — it made him feel old and tired, and every time he looked in the mirror after his shower he couldn't help but focus on his bulging belly. Driving to work one day, he noticed a medical antiaging clinic and decided to check it out. He had heard about testosterone supplements and wanted to see if they could boost his energy and libido and possibly trim that fat around his belly. After a brief clinic visit, he left with a two-month supply of pills.

Phil noticed results right away — he lost some weight and had more energy when he worked out, both on the treadmill and bench-pressing weights. His wife, Beverly, started noticing it too.

"You kept worrying that 60 was so old, but you seem younger since your birthday." She smiled slyly. "You certainly had a lot of energy last night in the bedroom."

As he continued to take the supplement, Phil enjoyed his improved strength, higher energy levels, and slimmer waistline, but he started having trouble sleeping at night. He kept waking up to urinate, and sometimes it hurt. He started to worry about side effects and finally discussed his testosterone use with his doctor.

After a checkup, Phil's doctor told him that his urinary frequency and pain was from an enlarged prostate. The good news was that his blood test was negative for cancer, but Phil needed to back off the testosterone. He took the doctor's advice, gave up the testosterone, and started sleeping better at night.

Like many men, Phil tried testosterone to fight off the effects of aging, but he had no clue of the potential dangers. In healthy men, testosterone levels peak at age 30 and then steadily decline by 1 to 2 percent each year. These drops can lower sex drive, mood, and energy, but men don't need supplementation unless their levels drop below 300 nanograms per deciliter. Because of the potential side effects, always check with your doctor first to determine if testosterone therapy is indicated. Although testosterone supplementation can improve mood and physical stamina, it can also cause enlarged prostate, blood clots from increased red blood cell counts, sleep apnea, liver damage, and prostate cancer.

testosterone still use the hormone, a risky business since testosterone can stimulate prostate cancer growth and increase the risk for a heart attack or stroke. Animal studies have demonstrated the potential brain-boosting effects of testosterone, and small-scale human trials have shown both cognitive improvement and worsening from intramuscular testosterone injections. Larger clinical studies are still needed to prove a true testosterone benefit for memory performance and brain health.

Dietary Supplements

Up to two-thirds of Americans take dietary supplements, and surveys suggest that supplement users tend to live healthy lifestyles by exercising, avoiding cigarettes, and eating nutritious diets. Regulations for approval of a vitamin, mineral, or other dietary supplement are less stringent than those for drugs. The 1994 Dietary Supplement and Health Education Act set forth the standards for manufacturers and distributors, prohibiting them from marketing poor quality or misbranded products. Manufacturers need to evaluate the safety and labeling of their products before marketing them to ensure they meet all regulatory requirements.

The consumer faces challenges in figuring out which supplements really work, what side effects to watch out for, and when drugs and supplements may interact and pose health risks. Potential hazards range from liver damage to excess bleeding and pain. Taking the popular memory supplement ginkgo biloba and drinking coffee could cause subdural hematomas (blood clots surrounding the brain), and ginkgo can influence the effects of insulin secretion, which could make it harmful for diabetics.

Taking large doses of some vitamins can have side effects. High doses of vitamins A, D, E, and K should be avoided because they are fat-soluble and stored in the body's fat cells, leading to potentially harmful buildups over time.

Concerns about risks and limited evidence of the brain benefits of supplements have led some experts to question whether

---

Too Much Calcium May Hurt Your Heart

Many women use daily calcium supplements to protect their bone health and lower their risk for developing osteoporosis, a medical condition that causes brittle and fragile bones. Lack of estrogen from menopause contributes to osteoporosis, but the US Preventive Services Task Force recently advised against calcium supplementation in postmenopausal women due to lack of scientific evidence demonstrating that it works to prevent the disease.

Not everyone knows that calcium supplements can lead to as much as 30 percent higher risk of a heart attack in women, as well as cardiovascular disease in both women and men. Excess calcium in the bloodstream may lead to deposits in arteries causing heart problems.

According to the Institute of Medicine, the recommended daily consumption is 1,000 milligrams for men ages 19 to 70 and women 19 to 50 (1,200 for older women). A safe and effective way to ingest enough calcium is through diet: 8 ounces of milk or 6 ounces of yogurt each contain about 300 milligrams of calcium. Other calcium-rich foods include canned salmon, sardines, kale, almonds, and broccoli.

---

we should be taking them at all. However, recent studies suggest promise for several dietary supplements that may improve brain health as we age. When deciding on which form of supplement to take, it's important to get accurate information about the brand reliability, effectiveness, and potential side effects. In addition to a knowledgeable pharmacist or physician, information is available from the National Center for Complementary and Integrative Health (www.nccih.nih.gov).

ANTIOXIDANT SUPPLEMENTS

Oxidative stress attacks the brain as it ages, causing wear and tear on cells, and antioxidant vitamins have been used to counteract the damage. In the late 1990s, a large-scale study showed that 2,000 units of vitamin E taken daily slowed the progression of Alzheimer's disease.

In 2005, other research indicated an association between taking 400 or more daily units of vitamin E and serious cardiac side effects, as well as increased risk of death. These potential side effects of high-dose vitamin E occurred in older individuals with previous heart disease, and a newer investigation supports the brain benefits of vitamin E for mild to moderate Alzheimer's disease. After more than two years of follow-up, the scientists found that patients receiving high-dose vitamin E experienced slower decline in daily functioning than those on a placebo. And, the patients taking vitamin E in this new study did not develop heart problems. Even though vitamin E may benefit patients with mild to moderate Alzheimer's disease, we still don't know whether it can delay the onset of Alzheimer's in people with normal aging.

Laboratory and animal studies point to potential cognitive benefits of the antioxidant supplements acetyl-l-carnitine and coenzyme Q10, but their ability to boost brain health in humans is not clear. Studies of vitamin C and beta-carotene have not shown consistent brain-protective results. Our initial UCLA work with pomegranate juice, which contains powerful polyphenol antioxidants, indicated cognitive improvements in people with mild memory changes, and larger-scale studies of the memory effects of pomegranate capsules and juice are ongoing.

Curry In A Pill

The prevalence of Alzheimer's disease appears to be lower in India compared with the United States and Europe, and curcumin (the active ingredient in turmeric) may protect the brains of millions of Indians who regularly consume curried foods. Although such statistics do not prove that eating Indian food will keep your brain young, laboratory studies have demonstrated anti-inflammatory, anti-amyloid, and antioxidant brain-boosting effects of curcumin.

If Indian food is not your thing, then stay tuned for clinical trials to determine if curcumin capsules work better than a placebo. Although initial research was negative in patients who already suffered from dementia, our UCLA group is conducting a double-blind, placebo-controlled study to determine whether curcumin capsules can delay memory decline and the buildup of plaques and tangles in the brain in people at risk for dementia.

B AND D VITAMINS

Not everyone absorbs adequate amounts of vitamin B, so these vitamins are usually included in multivitamin supplements. Folate, or folic acid (an antioxidant B vitamin), may protect older adults from developing strokes and heart disease, but too much folate may impair memory in older people who have low vitamin B12 levels. Vitamins B6, B12, and folate are involved in the breakdown of homocysteine (an amino acid building block of protein), and high homocysteine blood levels increase the risk for Alzheimer's disease. Oxford University scientists found that two years of vitamin B supplementation in patients with mild cognitive impairment slowed cognitive decline and brain shrinkage compared with a placebo. Vitamin B12 also may boost brain health by controlling inflammation.

Sunlight and milk products provide vitamin D, but many people spend too much time indoors and are deficient in this vitamin. Low vitamin D levels are associated with cognitive decline, and a study of approximately 5,000 older women showed that those taking the recommended weekly amount had better cognitive function than those who did not, but not all studies have replicated such benefits.

OMEGA-3 SUPPLEMENTS

Two essential omega-3 fatty acids, eicosapentaenoic acid (EPA) and docosahexaenoic acid (DHA), are necessary for normal brain development. The scientific evidence suggests that dietary omega-3 fats fight brain inflammation and boost memory as well as mood. People who consume omega-3 fatty acids have a lower risk of cognitive decline as they get older, but many people do not get enough dietary omega-3 fats.

Omega-3 supplements have not helped patients who already have dementia, but they may offer a benefit for people with only mild age-related memory complaints. A 2012 study of healthy adults aged 50 to 75 showed that a daily 2.2-gram omega-3 supplement taken for a four-month period led to significant improvements in cognitive abilities compared with a placebo. People with higher levels of omega-3 fat have larger brains, especially in their hippocampal memory centers. Omega-3s also improve executive function, which translates into better planning, organization, and management skills.

GINKGO BILOBA

Ginkgo is a popular supplement that many people take to improve their memory and mental focus. This antioxidant supplement increases brain circulation and enhances the absorption of sugar into brain cells. Possible side effects include upset stomach, dizziness, headache, bleeding, and lowering of blood pressure. Some studies have demonstrated positive memory effects of ginkgo in people with normal aging. However, a recent six-year study of more than 3,000 older adults showed that 120 milligrams of ginkgo taken twice a day was no better than a placebo in slowing cognitive decline in both normal aging and mild cognitive impairment.

HUPERZINE A

Many of the drugs available to treat Alzheimer's dementia increase the availability of the brain messenger acetylcholine in order to stimulate neuron function. Huperzine A is a dietary supplement that is thought to work the same way. Some studies have demonstrated its effectiveness in patients with dementia as well as milder cognitive problems, but others show no benefits. A limited Chinese study indicated cognitive benefits in adolescents treated over a one-month period. Additional research is needed to demonstrate whether huperzine A improves memory abilities in people with mild age-related symptoms.

PHOSPHATIDYLSERINE

Phosphatidylserine plays a role in cellular communication and normal functioning of the lining around brain cells, and several

Healthcare for a Better Brain

- Partner with your doctor to address your health concerns and answer your questions about medical issues and lifestyle habits that affect your health.
- Bring all your medicines (or a list of them) to your doctor appointment to make sure that your prescription and over-the-counter drugs are not causing any memory side effects, and always discuss anything new you want to start taking.
- If you have high blood pressure or cholesterol, diabetes, or another chronic medical illness, your doctor's suggestions may be crucial for optimal brain health.
- Patients with Alzheimer's dementia can temporarily benefit from anti-dementia medicines that help maintain a higher level of functioning longer.
- Hormones and supplements have been used to treat age-related memory loss, but long-term benefits have not been confirmed.

studies suggest it may improve cognitive abilities. An investigation of 157 older people with mild memory complaints showed that phosphatidylserine plus an omega-3 fatty acid improved their memory compared with a placebo after 15 weeks of treatment. Several other investigations have demonstrated comparable benefits in similar study populations after 12 weeks of phosphatidylserine treatment without additional omega-3 fatty acid supplementation. These results are encouraging, but additional studies would be needed to prove benefits beyond three months of treatment.

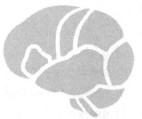

CHAPTER NINE

The 2-Week Younger Brain Program

"I not only use all the brains that I have, but all that I can borrow."

—*Woodrow Wilson*

B Y AGE 40, NEARLY everyone begins to experience a mild decline in their mental acuity. You might have trouble coming up with the name of a person you just met; perhaps you have to consult the owner's manual again to reset the clock in your car; or maybe you just opened the refrigerator and forgot what you were looking for. We can't stop the years from passing, but we can start taking action to keep our brains young. This chapter will provide a step-by-step guide to my two-week program that is easy to follow and designed to meet your personal brain health needs.

The goal is to alter your behavior and create new brain-healthy habits for the rest of your life. For a younger brain program to succeed in the long run, it must deliver three essential elements: knowledge of how your actions affect your brain, achievable milestones, and encouraging feedback along the way.

Knowledge Is Power

In the previous chapters of this book, you have seen the clear connection between your everyday lifestyle habits and your brain health. Your daily decisions on whether to exercise your mind and body, what you eat, and how you cope with stress have a direct effect on your brain age. Research has shown that when people understand this connection, they are more motivated to commit to a healthy lifestyle program and enjoy positive results for years.

Achievable Milestones

A common mistake that many health, diet, and exercise programs make is they set unreasonably high goals. (Lose 30 pounds in a month! Look five years younger overnight!) Because these goals are not realistic, people either give up on the program quickly or never even take it seriously.

Is two weeks to a younger brain promising too much? Not according to systematic scientific studies and the experience of thousands of people who have benefited from my methods. Also, my exercises start out easy, and you increase the challenge at your own pace, which allows you to easily achieve the milestones.

Feedback

Positive feedback encourages us to stay on track. If I go on a diet and my pants get looser around the waist, it makes me want to continue with my diet. When I step on the scale and see that I've lost five pounds, it increases my motivation even more. The 2-Week Younger Brain Program will bring quick and noticeable results: the brain aerobics will improve your memory and mental acuity, the physical exercise will give you more energy, the stress-reduction techniques will relax you, and the healthy-brain diet will boost your metabolism and help you lose unwanted weight. To reinforce this subjective feedback, I have built in brief quizzes for you to take on day 1, day 7, and day 14, which will measure your results and document them in black and white.

Building Brain Synergy

You will learn targeted strategies for all of the components of the program — mental training, physical exercise, stress management, and healthy nutrition — each of which helps keep your brain young. However, our UCLA research showed that when you combine these various strategies and practice them together, you create a synergy that gives the whole program a faster and greater impact.

In our UCLA collaborations with the Gallup Poll organization, we evaluated responses from more than 18,000 adults age 18 to 99 on several of the lifestyle strategies that comprise my two-week program. We found that the more strategies (e.g., physical exercise,

---

Your Brain-Healthy Diet

Changing how you eat to keep your brain young involves following a few guidelines:

- **Eat small meals throughout the day.** Have breakfast, a mid-morning snack, lunch, a mid-afternoon snack, and dinner to avoid getting too hungry at any one time.
- **Combine healthy proteins and carbohydrates at every meal.** This combination provides immediate energy from the carbs and sustained satiety from the proteins.
- **Get adequate hydration, vitamins, and minerals.** Drink several 8-ounce glasses of water, along with 1 multivitamin and 1,000 milligrams of omega-3 fatty acid (fish oil) each day.
- **Eat healthy omega-3 fats.** Eat fish at least twice each week and/or nuts and flaxseed to help control inflammation.
- **Include antioxidant fruits and vegetables.** Colorful fruits and green leafy vegetables fight oxidation and provide fiber to promote digestion.
- **Minimize omega-6 fats, refined sugars, and processed foods.** A steak or cookie once in a while is okay, but don't make a habit of it.
- **Practice portion control.** Try splitting entrées at restaurants and putting less on your plate at home.

healthy diet, not smoking) that people engaged in, the better their memory. Respondents who engaged in just one healthy behavior were 21 percent less likely to report a memory problem compared to those who didn't engage in any healthy behaviors. Those who engaged in three healthy behaviors were 75 percent less likely to notice any memory difficulties. Other studies have demonstrated the synergistic benefits of blending healthy behaviors in reducing the risk for diabetes and symptoms of heart disease.

The following are some examples of healthy meals:

Breakfast Suggestions

- Vegetable omelet (1 whole egg plus 2 egg whites mixed with such vegetables as spinach or peppers); ½ cup fresh or frozen blueberries; 1 slice whole-grain toast with natural jam

- ¾ cup hot oatmeal with 1 tablespoon raisins; ½ cup nonfat milk or yogurt; ½ grapefruit

- 8 ounces of yogurt with berries; ½ cup granola or 1 slice whole-grain toast

- Scrambled eggs (1 whole egg plus 2 egg whites) with 2 strips of turkey bacon; 1 slice wheat or rye toast with natural fruit jam; ½ cup fresh or frozen berries

Lunch

- Tuna sandwich (made with light mayo) on whole-grain bread, with lettuce and tomato; 1 cup grapes

- Grilled turkey dog on rye toast with mustard (sauerkraut optional); crisp apple

- Garden salad with 3–6 ounces grilled chicken or salmon; vinaigrette (balsamic vinegar and olive oil) dressing; 2 whole-grain crackers; orange sections

- Bowl of chicken soup (with white meat and vegetables); ½ toasted pita bread; sliced pear

Dinner

- You may include one glass of wine, beer, or a cocktail if you wish with any of the following meals:

- Grilled 6-ounce chicken breast with herbs; tossed green salad with vinaigrette dressing; ½ cup brown rice; steamed spinach; fruit sorbet (dessert)

- 4–6 ounce grilled salmon filet with herbs and lemon slices; tomato, avocado, and sweet onion salad drizzled with olive oil and lemon; boiled red potatoes; steamed broccoli; sliced fresh apple with cinnamon (dessert)

- Turkey burger on toasted whole-grain bun; spinach salad with chopped apple and walnuts with vinaigrette dressing; steamed spinach and carrots; fruit or frozen juice bar (dessert)

- 4–6 ounce lean steak; arugula and shaved Parmesan cheese salad tossed in vinaigrette dressing; steamed zucchini rounds; sliced strawberries with a scoop of frozen yogurt (dessert)

Snacks

- ½ cup yogurt with ½ banana

- Selection of raw vegetables (e.g., celery, red bell pepper, tomatoes); 1 ounce string cheese

- 1 cup tomato soup or juice; 1–2 ounces (up to ¼ cup) unsalted almonds or walnuts

- ½ cup low-fat cottage cheese, plus 1 tablespoon raisins mixed in

More Nutrition Tips

Although switching up your menus makes sense, some people do prefer certain dishes, so don't fret if you like the same
egg whites and toast with black coffee for breakfast every day.
The overall goal is to keep your diet nutritious and delicious.
Varying your entrées and snacks throughout the day and
week will make each meal more interesting and appealing.
Use spices liberally to enhance flavor and provide additional
antioxidant boosts.

Moderation is essential when it comes to portion size, caffeine
use, and alcohol consumption. Try to remain mindful of your
feelings of hunger and satisfaction throughout the day — that's
your body's natural feedback system helping you to achieve your
ideal body weight.

Vegetarians and Vegans

If you are a vegetarian or vegan, you can modify your nutrition
plan to accommodate your personal dietary choices. Vegetarian
diets exclude meat, poultry, and fish, while vegans also avoid
dairy products and eggs. Vegetarian diets usually include plenty
of carbohydrates and dietary fiber but are sometimes relatively
low in protein, vitamin B12, and omega-3 fats. Vegans need to
be careful to get enough protein, vitamin B12, and calcium from
their diets. Good sources of protein for vegetarians and vegans
include nuts, quinoa, tofu, lentils, beans, and tempeh. Taking
daily supplements helps ensure consumption of adequate brain-
healthy nutrients.

Physical Fitness

The program's physical conditioning, strength training, stretching, and balance exercises are safe for most people, but you may
wish to consult your doctor before starting. If you scored well
on your Baseline Physical Fitness questionnaire (chapter 6), you
may want to increase the intensity or repetitions of the exercises

in your program. You can also adjust any of the exercises in the book and add your own. If you already swim 40 laps or spend 45 minutes on the treadmill every day, your cardiovascular fitness is already good, but you may still need to focus on balance and strength training. Some of the exercises require an elastic band, which you can purchase at a local drugstore, sporting goods store, or online.

Walking is one of the safest and most efficient aerobic workouts. Studies have shown that 15 minutes of brisk walking a day (90 minutes a week) may be all you need to delay cognitive decline and reduce your risk for developing Alzheimer's disease. Walking with a friend compounds its benefits by adding the social connection and stress reduction you get from a good conversation.

The goal is to reach a total of 20 to 30 minutes of daily physical exercise. You can augment your fitness by melding exercise into your daily activities. For example, park or get dropped off a few minutes from your destination and walk the rest of the way, or choose the stairs over the elevator, at least for a few flights.

Mental Aerobics

The program's mental exercises are designed to become more challenging as you progress so you will gradually build brainpower and proficiency. If you find an exercise particularly difficult, repeat that exercise the following day before moving on. If an exercise is too easy for you, modify it to make it more challenging. For example, if I ask you to memorize four words, add a fifth one of your own choosing.

The aim of these next two weeks is to experience quick and easy results that create and reinforce brain-healthy habits. Behaviors become habits more readily when they are performed in consistent settings and at regular times. See the next page for your One-Minute Memory Test.

One-Minute Test to Rate Your Memory

Before you begin The 2-Week Younger Brain Program, take this quick memory test to assess your baseline abilities. Study the following 10 words for one minute and then put the book down and do something else for five minutes. After the five minutes, write down all the words you can remember without looking at the book. Afterward, compare your list with the actual list in the book and write your score in the box.

Shark	Harp
Leg	Street
Teacher	Wrench
Ink	Coffee
Lettuce	Newspaper

Now put down the book and follow the directions above.

BASELINE MEMORY SCORE: _____

Don't worry if you only remembered a few words; the 14-Day Younger Brain Program will boost your memory quickly, and you're bound to see an improved score next time.

The 2-Week Program

You're now ready to begin the program. On the following pages, you'll see the recommended exercises for each of the next 14 days. Try them at the suggested times (morning, afternoon, and evening) or find space in your schedule that may be more convenient for you. Take your time and enjoy yourself. You're only two weeks away from a younger brain.

DAY 1 MORNING

PHYSICAL FITNESS:

Side bend (stretch). Stand with your feet shoulder-width apart and hold your arms out to your sides. Lean to your left, reaching your right arm over your head until you feel a good stretch in your right side muscles. Hold for a count of five, and then switch to the other side. Repeat three times on each side.

Russian folk dance (conditioning). Stand up straight and fold your arms in front at shoulder height like a Russian folk dancer. Raise your right knee toward your right elbow, and then alternate, bringing your left knee up toward your left elbow. Repeat for a total of eight knee lifts with each leg.

BRAIN TRAINING:

FOCUS practice. Because you need to FOCUS your attention on new information before you can FRAME it with meaning, start with this warm-up exercise to improve your mental focus. Before you leave the house today, pay attention to an article of clothing that your spouse or roommate is wearing. It could be a blouse, shirt, tie, or jacket. Notice the colors, patterns, and texture. Jot down four details about it. If you live alone, focus on the clothing of the first person you encounter in the morning.

AFTERNOON

STRESS MANAGEMENT:

Muscle relaxation (meditation). Lie down or sit in a chair, take a few deep breaths, and then close your eyes. Pay attention to your forehead and scalp muscles. Release any tension there. Let the sense of relaxation spread down your face to your jaw muscles. Next, relax your neck and shoulder muscles (move them around a bit if it helps to relax them). Continue to breathe deeply and slowly as you gradually relax your upper and then lower body. Systematically relax all your muscles down to your toes. Enjoy this relaxed state for a moment before opening your eyes.

BRAIN TRAINING:

On the other hand. Warm up your neural circuits by practicing your signature with your nondominant hand (left hand if you are right-handed). Penmanship doesn't count today.

Brain games. Do a crossword, Sudoku, KenKen, or any other puzzle or computer brain game (see appendix 1 for brain game websites).

EVENING

PHYSICAL FITNESS:

Evening walk. Take a 10-minute walk before or after dinner. If circumstances do not permit a walk, repeat this morning's physical fitness routine.

BRAIN TRAINING:

Recall practice. Think about that piece of clothing you focused on this morning. Without using your notes, try to recall the four details. Check your notes to see how many details you remembered.

DAY 2 MORNING

PHYSICAL FITNESS:

Side bend. Hold for a count of five, and then switch to the other side. Repeat four times on each side.

Russian folk dance. Repeat for a total of 10 knee lifts with each leg.

BRAIN TRAINING:

FOCUS practice. Before leaving the house, repeat yesterday's FOCUS exercise but without written notes this time. Again, pay attention to an article of clothing on the first person you encounter, and notice colors, patterns, textures, and other features. After focusing on it, close your eyes. Imagine the item and think about the details.

Prospective memory habits. People often complain about forgetting appointments or things they intended to do or bring with them — activities that require prospective memory skills. Panic can set in when they get halfway to their destination and suddenly start worrying whether they've forgotten to close the garage door or left something important at home.

To avoid such incidents and boost your prospective memory skills, create a morning memory habit: Every day, at the same time and place, review your calendar and *all* your appointments before leaving the house. Think through the details of each appointment and plan. If you are going to the gym, don't forget your gym bag. Meeting with your accountant? Be sure to bring your paperwork. Finally, before you turn on your car ignition or head to the bus stop, run through a mental checklist of routine household matters: Did you turn off the stove? Lock the front door? Close the garage door?

AFTERNOON

STRESS MANAGEMENT:

Breathing (meditation). Lie down or sit in a comfortable position. Breathe slowly through your nose. Focus on your abdomen, expanding it with each inhale, and then slowly exhale as much air as possible. Feel your diaphragm rise and fall as you breathe. Spend two minutes focusing on your breathing.

BRAIN TRAINING:
FRAME practice. You have been working on paying attention to detail (FOCUS). Today you will practice FRAME — the ability to put those details into a context that makes them meaningful and memorable. These exercises build on your brain's innate hardwiring to remember visual images. You can train this skill when you purposely create memorable mental pictures.

For each of the following words, generate a visual image in your mind and make it more memorable by giving it vivid color and detail (e.g., instead of just imagining a rose, envision a bright red rose with a thorny stem and dew drops):

Rose
Poodle
Oven
Kite

EVENING

PHYSICAL FITNESS:
Evening walk. Take a 10-minute walk before or after dinner. If circumstances do not permit a walk, repeat this morning's physical fitness routine.

BRAIN TRAINING:
Recall practice. Try to recall the details of the clothing you focused on this morning. No notes this time — simply close your eyes and see if that helps you remember more details. Now try to remember the four items that you practiced visualizing this afternoon.

DAY 3 MORNING

PHYSICAL FITNESS:

Side bend. Repeat four times on each side.

Chest stretch. Stand straight and clasp your hands low behind your back. Keeping your chest high, lift your straight arms up and out behind you. Feel the stretch in your chest as you hold for five seconds and then repeat.

Russian folk dance. Repeat for a total of 10 knee lifts on each side.

BRAIN TRAINING:

Memory habits. Check your calendar before leaving the house: remember to do it at the same time and same place every day to form a good memory habit. Review your house-closing routines before leaving for the day.

Names and faces. If you're like most people, you don't always remember people's names and faces. You can use the FOCUS and FRAME method to improve this important everyday memory skill. Meet Professor Baldwin and take about 30 seconds (probably much longer than you'd spend in a typical social situation) to study his name and face.

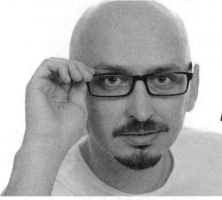

Professor Baldwin

AFTERNOON

STRESS MANAGEMENT:

Muscle relaxation. This time spend three minutes relaxing the major muscle groups in your body.

Talking and listening (also see chapter 7). Improving your ability to listen to partners and friends will improve those relationships and lower stress levels. Focus on feelings and avoid criticism during this exercise. Set your timer for two minutes and ask your partner to discuss any problem, issue, or challenge he or she is experiencing. As you listen, maintain eye contact and do not interrupt. After your two minutes of listening, reset the timer for two minutes and this time you speak while your partner listens. After the two minutes, take turns discussing how you felt about the exercise.

BRAIN TRAINING:

Memory practice. Keeping your brain young involves optimizing its cognitive efficiency. To avoid wasting mental energy remembering where you put commonly misplaced objects, create memory places for your things. For example, keys can go on a hook by the door; glasses on your bedside table. If you haven't created them already, come up with memory places for these items: eyeglasses, medicine, wallet, scissors, checkbook, and cell phone. Use FOCUS and FRAME to memorize your new memory places.

EVENING

PHYSICAL FITNESS:

Evening walk. Take a 10-minute walk before or after dinner.

BRAIN TRAINING:

FOCUS and FRAME practice. To continue to strengthen your FOCUS and FRAME skills, memorize the following word pairs by creating images in your mind that link each pair together. For example, to link the words "nurse — toast," you might visualize a nurse eating a piece of toast, or perhaps she is toasting her best friend at a wedding. Take up to two minutes to FOCUS on and then FRAME the following unrelated word pairs:

Chimes — Horse
Door — Airplane
Elevator — Bracelet

DAY 4 MORNING

 PHYSICAL FITNESS:

Side bend. Repeat five times on each side.

Chest stretch. Hold for five seconds and repeat three times.

Russian folk dance. Repeat for a total of 15 knee lifts on each side.

 BRAIN TRAINING:

Memory habits. Don't forget your new memory habit of checking your calendar and routines before leaving the house.

Recall practice. See if you can remember last night's word pairs. Below are the first words of each pair. See how quickly you can recall the second word of each pair (use your visual brain to concentrate on the images you created last night).

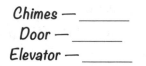

Chimes — _____
Door — _____
Elevator — _____

Do you remember the name of the guy I introduced you to yesterday? What were his distinguishing features? How did you link his name to his face? Did you see his **bald** head or picture him **win**ning at poker? Was he giving a lecture and using his eyeglasses to point at the blackboard like a ***professor***?

AFTERNOON

STRESS MANAGEMENT:
Breathing. Spend three minutes on this exercise today. Focus on your abdomen moving as you inhale and exhale.

Get Realistic. Many of us are stressed out because we take on too many tasks. Make a list of things you plan to do in the next two days and see if you can skip, delegate, or postpone any nonurgent tasks. Perhaps ask a friend, family member, or coworker to help out.

BRAIN TRAINING:
Noticing details. Create a visual image in your mind for each of the places below, and list three details you might see in each image:

Schoolyard: _____, _____, _____

Racetrack: _____, _____, _____

Circus: _____, _____, _____

EVENING
PHYSICAL FITNESS:
Evening walk. Take a 15-minute walk before or after dinner.

BRAIN TRAINING:

Names and faces. Meet my friend Eileen Bengal. Try to remember her name and face. As you do, you might notice her pretty eyes and her bangs.

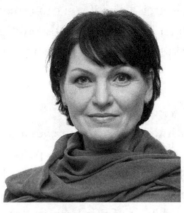

Eileen Bengal

Extra credit. Have fun with a crossword, Sudoku, Ken-Ken, or any other puzzle or computer brain game to keep your neural circuits limber.

DAY 5 MORNING

PHYSICAL FITNESS:

Side bend. Repeat five times on each side.

Chest stretch. Hold for five seconds and repeat three times.

Russian folk dance. Repeat for a total of 15 knee lifts on each side.

The flamingo (balance practice). While standing, focus on a point in front of you (e.g., a painting on a wall, a book on a shelf). Next, lift your right foot off the floor — if you need to, outstretch your arms to help you balance. Hold for a count of five and then switch to the other side.

BRAIN TRAINING:
Memory habits. Check your calendar and routines before leaving the house.

Recall practice. Try to recall the three places from yesterday afternoon's exercise. See if you can remember all three details for each place. Clue: you would probably prefer to take your kids or grandkids to two of the places.

AFTERNOON

STRESS MANAGEMENT:
"On holiday" meditation. Close your eyes and imagine yourself in a relaxing holiday setting — perhaps you're lying on a tropical beach watching the waves or lounging by a glimmering pool at a desert resort. Breathe deeply as you imagine the details of this beautiful setting: the cool breeze, the warm sun, the feeling of sand between your toes. If other thoughts enter your mind, let them go and refocus your attention on your imaginary holiday. Continue vacationing for two minutes.

BRAIN TRAINING:
Right brain exercise. Here's a spatial exercise to keep your visual neural circuits flexible. Take five toothpicks and arrange them so they are all touching and display the number five.

Names and faces. Let's strengthen your ability for recalling names. For each of the following names, think of a visual image to help you remember it:

Dr. Lincoln
Mrs. Frank
Mr. Parker

By the way, do you remember the name of that woman you met yesterday? Hint: She had pretty eyes and bangs.

EVENING

PHYSICAL FITNESS:

Evening walk. Take a 15-minute walk before or after dinner.

BRAIN TRAINING:

Recall practice. Let's check your longer-term memory abilities. Do you remember the three places from your exercise yesterday? Clue: one of them is a place you might visit if you felt lucky.

Story method. Let's review how you can use FOCUS and FRAME to become proficient in the story method. Instead of just two unrelated words, you can connect three or more unrelated words by generating a brief story that links the words together. Here's a practical example: You have three errands tomorrow — buy tomatoes, repair a tire, and go to the bank. To remember all three, you might visualize yourself sitting on an old tire in front of a bank ATM as you juggle three tomatoes. To make it really memorable, one of the tomatoes could fall and splatter on your white shirt (this would work great if going to the cleaners was your fourth errand).

DAY 6 MORNING

PHYSICAL FITNESS:

Side bend. Repeat five times on each side.

Chest stretch. Hold for five seconds and repeat three times.

Twisting boxer (conditioning). Stand with feet apart, knees slightly bent, and arms by your sides. Twist your body to the left and push and throw a right punch toward the upper left corner of the room. Now reverse it and throw a left punch to the upper right corner of the room. Get in five punches on each side.

The flamingo. Hold for a count of five and then switch to the other side.

Bicep curl (strength training). Hold an end of your elastic band in each hand and stand on the center of the band. Start with your arms down by your sides and your palms facing forward. Now bend your forearms up toward your shoulders, keeping the band taut and your upper arms against your torso. Lower your forearms slowly and repeat four times.

 BRAIN TRAINING:
Memory habits. Don't forget to check your calendar and routines before leaving the house.

Toothpick puzzle. Let's continue yesterday's right brain exercise. Here is how your toothpicks should have been arranged so they are all touching and display the number five:

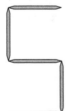

Now, rearrange the five toothpicks so they display an unlucky number.

Story method practice. Use FOCUS and FRAME plus the story memory method to memorize the following three words:

Duck   *Shoes*   *Umbrella*

AFTERNOON

STRESS MANAGEMENT:

Muscle relaxation. Spend five minutes relaxing the muscles throughout your body.

BRAIN TRAINING:

Names and faces. You just ran into the following two people at the supermarket. Do you remember their names?

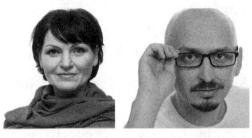

EVENING

PHYSICAL FITNESS:

Evening walk. Take a 15-minute walk before or after dinner.

BRAIN TRAINING:

Names and faces. Do you remember the visual images for the three names you learned yesterday afternoon? Hint: one could have been a bearded US president.

FRAME practice. When linking two images together to memorize unrelated words, keep in mind the following strategies to create more memorable associations:

» Use action to connect objects — one object may rotate or dance around the other, or perhaps they merge.

» Incorporate details into your images.

» Go with your first associations.

» Generate humorous or unusual imagery to make associations more memorable.

Here's an example: To remember a connection for the word pair "giraffe — window," imagine yourself awakened by a giraffe tapping on your upstairs bedroom window. He taps too hard, shatters the glass, and smiles as he tries to lick you.

DAY 7 MORNING

PHYSICAL FITNESS:
Side bend. Repeat five times on each side.

Russian folk dance. Repeat for a total of 20 knee lifts on each side.

Twisting boxer. Get five punches in on each side.

The flamingo. Hold for a count of 10 and then switch to the other side.

BRAIN TRAINING:
Memory habits. Fortify your prospective memory like you should every day: check your calendar and routines in the morning.

Recall practice. Do you remember the story you thought up yesterday to learn those three unrelated words? Perhaps your story took place on a rainy day.

Story method. Let's continue to build your story method abilities by creating a narrative that links the following four words:

Walrus   *Hammer*

Scooter   *Boy Scout*

AFTERNOON

STRESS MANAGEMENT:

Breathing. Take a five-minute break to breathe deeply through your nose. Feel your diaphragm rise and fall as you inhale and exhale.

Get realistic. Make a list of things you have to do in the next couple of days; postpone one nonurgent task and consider asking a friend or coworker to help out on one.

BRAIN TRAINING:

Names and faces. Some names are easy to visualize because they immediately bring an image to mind. You can see Mrs. **House** standing in front of her **house**. Others require more creativity. You might picture Mr. **Parker** in a valet uniform **parking** your car. (Didn't you see that name recently?)

Create visual images for the following four names:

Taylor

Paul

Joy

Misty

Recall practice. If I say "window," what unrelated word comes to mind? You remember, he was trying to lick you.

EVENING

PHYSICAL FITNESS:

Evening walk. Take a 15-minute walk before or after dinner.

BRAIN TRAINING:

On the other hand. Try signing your name with your non-dominant hand again, but this time penmanship counts.

Recall practice. See if you can recall the story you made up this morning. It should include a tool and something that children like to ride.

Do you remember the four names from yesterday afternoon? Hint: one might have been sewing a hem. Another might have been walking in the fog.

One-Week Memory Assessment

Great work! You're halfway through your two-week program, and you are probably noticing better mental focus, improved short-term memory, and increased energy levels. To prove to yourself that your brain is already younger than it was a week ago, repeat the objective assessment you performed at baseline, but with a new list of words.

Study the following 10 words for one minute. Then put the book aside and do something else for five minutes. After five minutes, write down as many words as you can remember.

Clown	*Crayon*
Ski	*Raft*
Piano	*Blanket*
Banana	*Book*
Artist	*Pencil*

I'm assuming your five minutes are up and you have written down on a separate piece of paper all the words you remembered.

Check the list above, write in your current score for the correct number of words that you recalled, and compare your current score to your baseline.

BASELINE MEMORY SCORE: _____

1 WEEK: _____

I suspect that you have improved by at least one or two points. That's an excellent sign that the program is boosting your brain health and helping you to create new habits. Solidifying those habits will be our goal for the next week.

DAY 8 MORNING

PHYSICAL FITNESS:

Side bend. Repeat six times on each side.

Chest stretch. Hold for five seconds and then repeat three times.

Russian folk dance. Repeat for a total of 20 knee lifts on each side.

Twisting boxer. Get eight punches in on each side.

The flamingo. Hold for a count of 15 and then switch to the other side.

Bicep curl. Repeat five times.

BRAIN TRAINING:

Memory habits. What are you supposed to remember to do today? Check your calendar first thing and see. Check your routine list before leaving the house.

Story method. You have graduated to advanced-placement story method. Create a story that includes all six of the following words:

Barn	*Aardvark*
Cigar	*Ottoman*
Tree	*Convertible*

AFTERNOON

STRESS MANAGEMENT:

"On holiday" meditation. Take five minutes to really enjoy your imaginary mini-vacation.

BRAIN TRAINING:
Word generation exercise. Get a pen and paper, and then make a list of as many animals that begin with the letter "P" as you can think of. (My list at end of the program.)

EVENING

 PHYSICAL FITNESS:
Evening walk. Take a 15-minute walk before or after dinner.

 BRAIN TRAINING:
Roman Room method: You've made it to the final few days of your program and are already a memory pro. Now I'd like you to use the ancient Roman Room method (see chapter 2) to memorize the names and order of the last five US vice presidents: Joe Biden, Dick Cheney, Al Gore, Dan Quayle, and George Bush. Get started with the following steps:

1. Imagine walking through five familiar rooms in your house along a fixed path.
2. Now take another mental stroll through your rooms along the same path, and visualize an image of one of the vice presidents in each room. For example, you might see Joe Biden biding time in your bedroom. (My images at end of chapter.)

DAY 9 MORNING

 PHYSICAL FITNESS:
Side bend. Repeat eight times on each side.

Russian folk dance. Repeat for a total of 20 knee lifts on each side.

Twisting boxer. Get eight punches in on each side.

The flamingo. Hold for a count of 15 and then switch to the other side.

Upper body pull-down (strength training). Stand with your feet wider than your shoulders and your toes pointing out. Gripping both ends of your resistance band, raise your arms overhead and move them outward to form a V as you pull the band taut. Stretch the band wider as you pull it down in front of your chest. Hold for a second and repeat three times.

BRAIN TRAINING:

Memory habits. Have you checked your daily calendar and routines?

Practice FOCUS and FRAME. Here are some more word pairs to memorize using FOCUS and FRAME. The challenge is increased because the words require more imagination in order to create images. For example, the word "idea" is a bit abstract. You can't actually see an idea, but you can visualize a light bulb appearing above your head signifying an idea.

Try to memorize these related word pairs, which include one abstract word and one more concrete (readily visualized) word.

Policeman — Speed
Lectern — Politics
Mountain — Steep

AFTERNOON

STRESS MANAGEMENT:

Mantra Meditation. Sit crossed-legged on the floor or in a comfortable chair. Close your eyes and breathe deeply and slowly. Concentrate on a single syllable or word of your choice, known as a mantra, while you inhale and exhale. If your mind wanders, simply bring your attention back to your mantra. Meditate for three minutes.

BRAIN TRAINING:

Tip of the Tongue. So far you've built skills to help master three of the four most common memory challenges: names and faces, memory places (where you put things), and prospective memory (appointments, plans, and routines). Now let's work on the fourth most common memory challenge, the tip-of-the-tongue phenomenon — where you know the word or name, it's on the tip of your tongue, but it just won't roll off.

You'll need to keep a paper and pencil handy at all times (techies can use their smartphones). The next time you have a tip-of-the-tongue experience, immediately write down any associations you can make to the word or name you can't quite remember. As soon as you get a chance, look up the information in a book or on the Internet, or ask someone who would know. Finally, use FOCUS and FRAME to link the associations you wrote down to the word that wouldn't roll off the tip of your tongue so that next time it will be easy to remember.

EVENING

PHYSICAL FITNESS:

Evening walk. Take a 20-minute walk before or after dinner.

BRAIN TRAINING

Story recall. Do you remember the story you made up yesterday so you could recall six unrelated words? Here are some clues: you might have seen an animal eating ants and someone driving with the top down.

Name recall. I've introduced you to several names and faces in the last nine days. Write down a list of the names you recall and count them up. (Nine is a perfect score by my count — see list at end of program.)

Narrative recall. Do you remember the narrative from chapter 2 about a woman who misplaced something? See the image below and describe what she misplaced and how she finally found it?

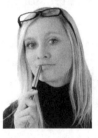

DAY 10 MORNING

PHYSICAL FITNESS:

Chest stretch. Hold for five seconds and then repeat three times.

Russian folk dance. Repeat for a total of 20 knee lifts on each side.

Twisting boxer. Get eight punches in on each side.

Heel-toe walk (balance). Stand with one foot in front of the other, heel to toe. Take 10 steps in that manner, touching the heel of your front foot to the toes of your back foot. Keep your eyes fixed on a point in front of you for added stability.

Bicep curl. Repeat eight times.

BRAIN TRAINING:

Memory habits. Check your calendar and routines this morning to boost your prospective memory.

Word-pair recall. Do you remember the word pairs from yesterday? They were related words. (My associations at the end of the program.)

AFTERNOON

STRESS MANAGEMENT:

Muscle Relaxation. Take five minutes to meditate and release your muscle tension.

BRAIN TRAINING

Remembering nonvisual names. When trying to remember a complicated name, or one that doesn't immediately bring an image to mind, try altering the name or its spelling slightly. To visualize the name Tyler, see her working as a tailor. For Paul, visualize him on top of a pole. Now alter these names so you can generate a visual image. (My suggestions at end of program.)

    Tom Siegel   *Olivia Newton*   *Rosa Flores*

EVENING

PHYSICAL FITNESS:

Evening walk. Take a 15-minute walk before or after dinner.

BRAIN TRAINING

Vice presidential recall. Do you still remember the last five US vice presidents? Mentally stroll through your rooms again and try to write them down in the correct order.

Seven-word story. Keep building your story method skills. Create a narrative to remember the following seven words, some related, some unrelated. (My story at end of program.)

| Window | Bed | Cloud | Pillow |
| Lightning | Spider | Cup | |

DAY 11 MORNING

PHYSICAL FITNESS:

Side bend. Repeat eight times on each side.

Chest stretch. Hold for five seconds; repeat three times.

Twisting boxer. Get eight punches in on each side.

The flamingo. Hold for a count of 15; switch sides.

Heel-toe walk. Take 10 steps.

Upper body pull-down. Repeat five times.

BRAIN TRAINING:

Memory habits. It's time for your morning calendar and routine check.

Observation exercise. Let's take another look at the photograph below from chapter 2. Focus on its details for 20 seconds and then cover the photo with a piece of paper.

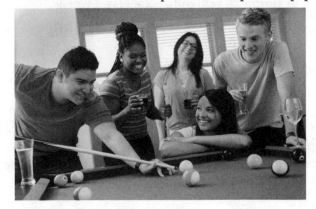

With the photo hidden, see if you can answer the following questions correctly:

» How many windows were in the photo?

» How many mugs or glasses? Were there any wine glasses?

» Did you notice the window treatments? What were they?

» How many people were touching the pool table?

AFTERNOON
STRESS MANAGEMENT:

Mantra Meditation. Concentrate on your mantra for a five-minute meditation.

BRAIN TRAINING:

Memorizing a new name. Your travel agent's assistant, *Sherry*, helps you with some travel arrangements. You want to make sure you remember her name the next time you call, but you have never seen her face so you can't focus on a distinguishing feature. You did note that she was very cheery. Next time you call the travel agency you'll remember to thank *cheery Sherry* (name altered slightly to make it more memorable).

Story recall. Try to recall the story you made up yesterday to remember the seven words.

EVENING
PHYSICAL FITNESS:

Evening walk. Take a 20-minute walk before or after dinner.

BRAIN TRAINING

Memorizing errands. Put the story method to use today. After checking your calendar and routines, write down a list of your appointments and errands. Use the FOCUS and FRAME method to create a story that will help you remember them. If you are really confident, leave the list at home and only use your story to remember your tasks.

Name recall. Do you recall the name of your travel agent's assistant? Remember how cheery she was?

DAY 12 MORNING

PHYSICAL FITNESS:

Side bend. Repeat eight times on each side.

Chest stretch. Hold for five seconds and then repeat three times.

Russian folk dance. Repeat for a total of 20 knee lifts on each side.

Heel-toe walk. Take 10 steps.

Bicep curl. Repeat 10 times.

BRAIN TRAINING

Word pairs. Use FOCUS and FRAME to learn the following word pairs:

Corn — Subway
Map — Watch
Escalator — Lizard

Meet and remember a new face. Practice your skill at learning names and faces. Make a point of meeting or introducing yourself to someone new today and use FOCUS and FRAME to learn their name and face. If you don't have a chance to meet someone, use a photo of someone in a magazine or newspaper.

AFTERNOON

STRESS MANAGEMENT:

Breathing Meditation. Time for another five-minute meditation break.

BRAIN TRAINING:

A Bogart tip-of-the-tongue. My wife continually forgets the name of a popular old Humphrey Bogart movie. Her associations are that it starred Humphrey Bogart and there was a bird in the title. She used those clues to look up the title, *The Maltese Falcon*. Use FOCUS and FRAME to create an image that would help my wife remember this title for good. (My answer at end of chapter.)

Remember her name and face. I'd like you to meet a young lady whose name is Franny. It's easy to remember her if you link her name to a distinguishing feature. (My association at end of chapter.)

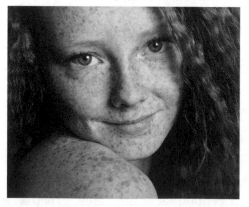

Franny

EVENING

PHYSICAL FITNESS:

Evening walk. Take a 20-minute walk before or after dinner.

BRAIN TRAINING:
Names and faces. Do you remember the new person you met yesterday? Make an attempt to meet someone new tomorrow and use FOCUS and FRAME to memorize their name and face

---

DAY 13 MORNING
 PHYSICAL FITNESS:
Chest stretch. Hold for five seconds and then repeat three times.

Twisting boxer. Get eight punches in on each side.

The flamingo. Hold for a count of 15 and then switch to the other side.

Upper body pull-down. Repeat eight times.

 BRAIN TRAINING:
Word-pair recall. Let's see how quickly you can recall the second word for each of yesterday's word pairs:

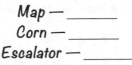

Map — _____
Corn — _____
Escalator — _____

Do you recall this young lady's name?

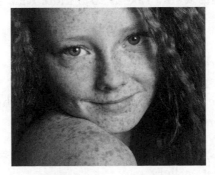

AFTERNOON

STRESS MANAGEMENT:

Mantra meditation. Take five minutes to release stress.

BRAIN TRAINING:

Name-face memory tips. Your ability to learn and re-call names and faces is likely impressive by now. In addition to using the FOCUS and FRAME method when you meet someone new, keep in mind the following tips to supercharge this skill:

1. When you meet someone new, repeat his or her name during the conversation.
2. If their name is unusual or complex, ask them to spell it and visualize the letters as you hear them. You can break up the syllables and create a visual image for each syllable.
3. Ask about details of their life and think about their name as they describe those details.
4. Do they remind you of anyone? Connecting a new person to someone you already know helps your hip-pocampus anchor the memory.

EVENING

PHYSICAL FITNESS:

Evening walk. Take a 20-minute walk before or after dinner.

BRAIN TRAINING:

Word generation exercise. Think of seven animals that begin with the letter "D" and jot them down. (My answers at the end of chapter.)

Let's see if you still remember the names of the people you met earlier:

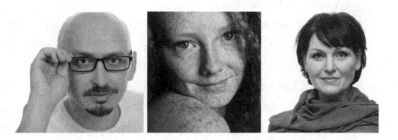

DAY 14 MORNING

 PHYSICAL FITNESS:

Side bend. Repeat eight times on each side.

Russian folk dance. Repeat for a total of 20 knee lifts on each side.

The flamingo. Hold for a count of 15 and then switch to the other side. Now try it with your eyes closed.

Bicep curl. Repeat 12 times.

 BRAIN TRAINING:

Memory habits. Check your calendar and routines before leaving the house. This is the last time I will remind you, I promise.

Keep your neural circuits tuned up by learning some more unrelated word pairs:

Calendar — Apple
Basketball — River
Jacket — Kite

AFTERNOON

 STRESS MANAGEMENT:

Meditation exercise of your choice. Five minutes.

BRAIN TRAINING:

Sorting exercise. When our brains organize information into categories, it makes it easier to remember. When I go to the market, I know it's easier to remember that I need to buy two cereals and two fruits rather than four items that are not sorted into categories. Strengthen your sorting skills by identifying the four categories for the following 16 items and then sort them into their proper categories:

Orange	Rugby	Sonata	Avocado
Tennis	Jazz	Apple	Dachshund
Grapes	Beagle	Track	Wrestling
Opera	Poodle	Terrier	Concerto

EVENING

PHYSICAL FITNESS:

Evening walk. Take a 20-minute walk before or after dinner.

BRAIN TRAINING:

Word-pair recall. Here are the first words of the word pairs you learned this morning. See how quickly you can recall the second word for each pair:

Calendar — _____
Basketball — _____
Jacket — _____

On the other hand. Have some fun tonight and try brushing or combing your hair with your left hand (if you are right-handed).

Two-Week Memory Assessment

Let's repeat the assessment you performed at the beginning and midway through the program. Study the following 10 words for one minute. Then put the book aside and do something else for five minutes. After five minutes, write down as many words as you can remember to get your score.

Study the following 10 words for one minute. Then put the book aside and do something else for five minutes. After five minutes, write down as many words as you can remember.

Scissors	*Owl*
Globe	*Watermelon*
Lamp	*Clock*
Surfer	*Champagne*
Computer	*Desk*

Two-Week Memory Score:
Now compare your three scores below:

    BASELINE MEMORY SCORE: _____

                1 WEEK: _____

            2 WEEKS: _____

I am confident that you did well on your final objective memory quiz. Keep up the good work and you'll enjoy a sharper memory, enhanced mental focus, better fitness, and overall well-being for years to come.

Congratulations!

You have completed your two-week program and you already have a younger brain! As you continue to practice your new healthy brain habits, they will become second nature in no time.

ANSWERS TO BRAIN TEASERS:
Page 214: Toothpick Puzzle.

Page 220: Word generation exercise.

"P" Animals: parakeet, parrot, partridge, peacock, pelican, penguin, pheasant, pigeon, platypus, porcupine, possum, puma, python.

Page 220: Roman Room method.

I visualize Joe **Biden** in my kitchen **biting** into a sandwich. As I walk down the hall, I pass Dick **Cheney** wearing a huge gold **chain**. I enter the den and find Al **Gore** watching a **gory** movie on TV. In the dining room, I see Dan **Quayle** dining on **quail**. Finally, in the living room I notice George **Bush** dressed as Moses confronting a burning **bush**.

Page 223: Name recall.

Professor Baldwin, Eileen Bengal, Dr. Lincoln, Mrs. Frank, Mr. Parker, Taylor, Paul, Joy, Misty.

Page 224: Word-pair recall.

- A **policeman** uses a radar gun to clock my **speed** as I race by in my car.
- A candidate is speaking about **politics** from behind a **lectern**.
- I am climbing a **steep mountain**.

Page 224: Remembering nonvisual names.

- For **Tom Siegel**, visualize him playing a **tom-tom** drum with a **seagull** on his shoulder.
- For **Olivia Newton**, see her eating a Fig **Newton** with an **olive** on top (or you could just imagine her singing with **Olivia Newton** John).
- I see **Rosa Flores** dropping a large vase of **roses** on the **floor**.

Page 224: Seven-word story.

I get into bed and see a **spider** on my **pillow**. I scoop it up with my tea**cup** and set it outside on the **window**sill just as a dark **cloud** bursts with **lightning** and thunder.

Page 228: A Bogart tip-of-the-tongue.
To remember *The Maltese Falcon*, my wife now envisions Bogart sharing a chocolate **malt** with a **falcon** on his shoulder, sipping from its own straw.

Page 228: Remember her name and face.
Franny's freckles make her memorable.

Page 230: Word generation.
"**D**" **Animals:** deer, dingo, dog, dolphin, donkey, dove, duck.

Page 232: Sorting exercise.
- **Sports:** rugby, tennis, wrestling, track
- **Dogs:** dachshund, beagle, poodle, terrier
- **Fruits:** orange, avocado, apple, grapes
- **Music:** sonata, jazz, opera, concerto

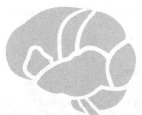

—APPENDIX ONE—

Brain Game Websites

"I am a brain, Watson. The rest of me is a mere appendix."

—*Arthur Conan Doyle*

BELOW YOU'LL FIND A list of websites offering free brain-building teasers, challenges, puzzles, and games for all ages.

- **Brain Den:** www.brainden.com

- **Brain Teasers:** www.brainteasers.org

- **BrainBashers:** www.brainbashers.com

- **Braingle:** www.braingle.com

- **Dakim BrainFitness:** www.dakim.com

- **Lumosity:** www.lumosity.com

- **PedagoNet:** www.pedagonet.com/brain/brainers.html

- **brainHQ:** www.brainhq.com

- **Sharp Brains:** www.sharpbrains.com

- **Syvum:** www.syvum.com/teasers

- **The Grey Labyrinth:** www.greylabyrinth.com

- **The Ultimate Puzzle Site:** www.puzzle.dse.nl

- **Tricky Riddles:** www.trickyriddles.com

- **Yahoo! Games:** www.games.yahoo.com

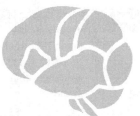

Additional Resources

"The chief function of the body is to carry the brain around."

—*Thomas A. Edison*

THERE IS NO SHORTAGE of resources geared toward the elderly population, especially as medicine and science continue to make groundbreaking discoveries in the areas of aging and brain research, and baby boomers mature into retirement at a rate of thousands per day. Consult the resources below in order to get yourself or a loved one on the road to healthful aging.

Name	Description	Telephone
AARP 6601 E Street NW Washington, DC 20049 www.aarp.org	Nonprofit that helps older Americans achieve independence, dignity, and purpose	888-687-2277
Administration for Community Living 1 Massachusetts Avenue NW Washington, DC 20001 www.acl.gov	Provides information for older Americans and their families to enrich their lives and support their independence	202-401-4634

Name	Description	Telephone
Alzheimer Europe 14 rue Dicks L-1417 Luxembourg www.alzheimer-europe.org	Organizes caregiver support and raises awareness about dementia in Europe	352-29-79-72
Alzheimer's Association 225 N. Michigan Avenue, Fl. 17 Chicago, IL 60611-7633 www.alz.org	Provides information on services, programs, publications, and local chapters	800-272-3900
Alzheimer's Foundation of America 322 Eighth Avenue, 7th floor New York, NY 10001 www.alzfdn.org	Supports organizations that improve quality of life of Alzheimer's patients and their caregivers	866-232-8484
Alzheimer's Disease Education & Referral Center PO Box 8250 Silver Spring, MD 20907 www.alzheimers.org	National Institute on Aging service that distributes information on topics relevant to professionals, patients and their families, and the general public	800-438-4380
American Academy of Neurology 201 Chicago Avenue Minneapolis, MN 55415 www.aan.com	Professional organization that advances the art and science of neurology and promotes the best possible care for patients with neurological disorders	800-879-1960
American Association for Geriatric Psychiatry 7910 Woodmont Avenue, #1050 Bethesda, MD 20814-3004 www.aagponline.org	Professional organization dedicated to enhancing the mental health and well-being of older adults through education and research	301-654-7850
American Geriatrics Society 40 Fulton Street, 18th Floor New York, NY 10038 www.americangeriatrics.org	Professional association providing assistance in identifying local geriatric physician referrals	212-308-1414 800-247-4779

Name	Description	Telephone
American Psychiatric Association 1000 Wilson Boulevard, Suite 1825 Arlington, VA 22209 www.psych.org	Medical specialty society that works to ensure humane care and effective treatment for people with mental disorders	888-357-7924
American Psychological Association 750 First Street NE Washington, DC 20002-4242 www.apa.org	Professional organization that represents US psychology and promotes health, education, and human welfare	800-374-2721
American Society on Aging 575 Market Street, Suite 2100 San Francisco, CA 94105-2869 www.asaging.org	National organization concerned with physical, emotional, social, economic, and spiritual aspects of aging	415-974-9600 800-537-9728
ClinicalTrials.gov www.clinicaltrials.gov	Registry of federal and private clinical trials with information on contacts, locations, and trial purposes	
Dana Alliance for Brain Initiatives 505 Fifth Avenue, 6th Floor New York, NY 10017 www.dana.org	Organization that advances public awareness about the progress and benefits of brain research	212-223-4040
Gerontological Society of America 1220 L Street NW, Suite 901 Washington, DC 20005 www.geron.org	National interdisciplinary organization on research and education in aging	202-842-1275
The Healthy Brain Initiative www.alz.org/publichealth/ downloads/2013-roadmap.pdf	A road map from the CDC and Alzheimer's Association to advance cognitive health as a vital, integral component of public health	
Monterey Bay Aquarium Seafood Watch www.seafoodwatch.org	Comparison of the mercury levels of different fish	

Name	Description	Telephone
National Center for Complementary and Integrative Health 9000 Rockville Pike Bethesda, MD 20892 www.nccih.nih.gov	The branch of the National Institutes of Health dedicated to exploring complementary and alternative healing practices in the context of rigorous science	888-644-6226
National Council on Aging 1901 L Street NW Washington, DC 20036 www.ncoa.org	A network of organizations and individuals dedicated to improving the health and independence of older persons and increasing their continuing contributions to society	202-479-1200
National Institute of Mental Health 6001 Executive Boulevard Bethesda, MD 20892 www.nimh.nih.gov	The branch of the National Institutes of Health that focuses on biomedical and behavioral research	301-443-8431 866-615-6464
National Institute of Neurological Disorders and Stroke PO Box 5801 Bethesda, MD 20824 www.ninds.nih.gov	The National Institutes of Health agency that supports neuroscience research; focuses on translating discoveries into prevention, treatment, and cures; and provides resource support and information	301-496-5751 800-352-9424
National Institute on Aging Building 31, Room 5C27 31 Center Drive, MSC 2292 Bethesda, MD 20892-2292 www.nih.gov/nia	One of the 27 institutes and centers of the National Institutes of Health; Primary federal agency supporting and conducting Alzheimer's disease research	301-496-1752 800-438-4380

Name	Description	Telephone
SeniorNet 5237 Summerlin Commons Boulevard Suite 314 Fort Myers, FL 33907 www.seniornet.com	National nonprofit organization that works to build a community of computer-using seniors	239-275-2202
UCLA Longevity Center 10945 Le Conte Avenue, #3119 Los Angeles, CA 90095-6980 www.aging.ucla.edu	University center that works to enhance and extend productive and healthy life through research and education on aging	310-794-0676
US Dept. of Veterans Affairs 810 Vermont Avenue NW Washington, DC 20420 www.va.gov	Provides information on VA programs, veterans' benefits, VA facilities worldwide, and VA medical automation software	800-827-1000

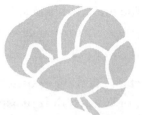

Bibliography

Chapter 1:
Brain-Boosting Discoveries for a Younger Mind

Small, G. W., et al. "Healthy behavior and memory self-reports in young, middle-aged, and older adults." *International Psychogeriatrics* 25, no. 6 (2013): 981–9.

Small, G. W., et al. "Effects of a 14-day healthy longevity lifestyle program on cognition and brain function." *American Journal of Geriatric Psychiatry* 14, no. 6 (2006): 538–45.

Merrill, D. A., and G. W. Small. "Prevention in psychiatry: effects of healthy lifestyle on cognition." *Psychiatric Clinics of North America* 34, no. 1 (2011): 249–61.

Sosa-Ortiz, A. L., et al. "Epidemiology of dementias and Alzheimer's disease." *Archives of Medical Research* 43, no. 8 (2012): 600–8.

Kaiser, N. C., et al. "The impact of age and Alzheimer's disease risk factors on memory performance over time." *Aging Health* 9, no. 1 (2013): 115–24.

Singh-Manoux, A., et al. "Timing of onset of cognitive decline: results from Whitehall II prospective cohort study." *British Medical Journal* 344 (2012): d7622. doi: 10.1136/bmj.d7622.

Brockmole, J. R., and R. H. Logie. "Age-related change in visual working memory: a study of 55,753 participants aged 8–75." *Frontiers in Psychology* 4, no. 12 (2013): 12.

Chen, S. T., et al. "Modifiable risk factors for Alzheimer disease and subjective memory impairment across age groups." *PLoS One* 4, no. 9: e98630. doi:10.1371/journal. pone.0098630.

Anguera, J. A., et al. "Video game training enhances cognitive control in older adults." *Nature* 501, no. 7465 (2013): 97–101.

Donix, M., et al. "APOE associated hemispheric asymmetry of entorhinal cortical thickness in aging and Alzheimer's disease." *Psychiatry Research* 214, no. 3 (2013): 212–20.

Ercoli, L.M., et al. "Perceived loss of memory ability and cerebral metabolic decline in persons with the apolipoprotein E-4 genetic risk for Alzheimer's disease." *Archives of General Psychiatry* 63, no. 4 (2003): 442–448.

Falk, D., et al. "The cerebral cortex of Albert Einstein: a description and preliminary analysis of unpublished photographs." *Brain* 136, pt. 4 (2013): 1304–27.

Bookheimer, S. Y., et al. "Patterns of brain activation in people at risk for Alzheimer's disease." *New England Journal of Medicine* 343, no. 7 (2000): 450–6.

Silverman, D. H. S., et al. "Positron emission tomography in evaluation of dementia: regional brain metabolism and long-term clinical outcome." *JAMA* 286, no. 17 (2001): 2120–7.

Small, G. W., et al. "PET of brain amyloid and tau in mild cognitive impairment." *New England Journal of Medicine* 355, no. 25 (2006): 2652–63.

Small, G. W., et al. "Prediction of cognitive decline by positron emission tomography of brain amyloid and tau." *Archives of Neurology* 69, no. 2 (2012): 215–2.

Braak, H., and E. Braak. "Neuropathological staging of Alzheimer-related changes." *Acta Neuropathologica* 82, no. 4 (1991): 239–59.

Small, G. W., et al. "Clinical, neuroimaging, and environmental risk differences in monozygotic female twins appearing discordant for dementia of the Alzheimer type." *Archives of Neurology* 50, no. 2 (1993): 209–19.

Head, D., et al. "Exercise engagement as a moderator of the effects of APOE genotype on amyloid deposition." *Archives of Neurology* 69, no. 5 (2012): 636–43.

Rowe, J. W., and R. L. Kahn. *Successful Aging.* New York: Dell Publishing, 1999.

Rowe, J. W., and R. L. Kahn. "The future of aging." *Contemporary Long-term Care* 22, no. 2 (1999): 36–8, 40, 42–44.

Corder, E. H., et al. "Gene dose of apolipoprotein E type 4 allele and the risk of Alzheimer's disease in late onset families." *Science* 261, no. 5123 (1993): 921–3.

Small, G. W., et al. "Cerebral metabolic and cognitive decline in persons at genetic risk for Alzheimer's disease." *Proceedings of the National Academy of Sciences of the United States of America* 97, no. 1 (2000): 6037–42.

Li, H., et al. "Molecular mechanisms responsible for
the differential effects of apoE3 and apoE4 on plasma
lipoprotein-cholesterol levels." *Arteriosclerosis, Thrombosis,
and Vascular Biology* 33, no. 4 (2013): 687–93.

Weinstein, G., et al. "Serum brain-derived neurotrophic factor
and the risk for dementia: the Framingham Heart Study."
JAMA Neurology 71, no. 1 (2014): 55–61.

Jonsson, T., et al. "Variant of TREM2 associated with the risk
of Alzheimer's disease." *New England Journal of Medicine*
368, no. 2 (2013): 107–16.

Small, G. W. "Paul McCartney's Memory Lapses." *HuffPost
Healthy Living*, August 27, 2010. http://www.huffingtonpost
.com/gary-w-small-md/paul-mccartneys-memory- la_b
_695560.html.

Gold, B. P., et al. "Pleasurable music affects reinforcement
learning according to the listener." *Frontiers in Psychology* 4
(2013): 541. doi: 10.3389/fpsyg.2013.00541.

Chan, M. F., et al. "Effects of music on depression in older
people: a randomized controlled trial." *Journal of Clinical
Nursing* 21, no. 5–6 (2012): 776–83.

Cross, K., et al. "The effect of passive listening versus active
observation of music and dance performances on memory
recognition and mild to moderate depression in cognitively
impaired older adults." *Psychological Reports* 111, no. 2
(2011): 413–23.

Green, A. C., et al. "Listen, learn, like! Dorsolateral prefrontal
cortex involved in the mere exposure effect in music."
Neurology Research International 2012: 846270. doi:
10.1155/2012/846270.

Bolla, K. I., et al. "Dose-related neurocognitive effects of marijuana use." *Neurology* 59, no. 9 (2002): 1337–43.

Scholes, K. E., and M. T. Martin-Iverson. "Cannabis use and neuropsychological performance in healthy individuals and patients with schizophrenia." *Psychological Medicine* 40, no. 10 (2010): 1635–46.

Morgan, C. J., et al. "Impact of cannabidiol on the acute memory and psychotomimetic effects of smoked cannabis: naturalistic study [corrected]." *British Journal of Psychiatry* 197, no. 4 (2010): 285–90.

Leuner, B., et al. "Sexual experience promotes adult neurogenesis in the hippocampus despite an initial elevation in stress hormones." *PLoS One* 5, no. 7 (2010): e11597.

Smith, G. D., S. Frankel, and J. Yarnell. "Sex and death, are they related? Findings from the Caerphilly cohort study." *British Medical Journal* 315, no. 7123 (1997): 1641–5.

Charnetski, C. J., and F. X. Brennan. "Sexual frequency and salivary immunoglobulin A (IgA)." *Psychological Reports* 94, no. 3, pt. 1 (2009): 839–44.

Ybarra, O., et al. "Mental exercising through simple socializing: social interaction promotes general cognitive functioning." *Personality and Social Psychology Bulletin* 34, no. 2 (2008): 248–59.

Lupien, S. J., et al. "Cortisol levels during human aging predict hippocampal atrophy and memory deficits." *Nature Neuroscience* 1, no. 1 (1998): 69–73.

Wilson, R. S., et al. "Proneness to psychological distress is associated with risk of Alzheimer's disease." *Neurology* 61, no. 11 (2003): 1479–85.

Pressman, S. D., and S. Cohen. "Does positive affect influence health?" *Psychological Bulletin* 131, no. 6 (2005): 925–71.

Acevedo, B. P., et al. "Neural correlates of long-term intense romantic love." *Social Cognitive and Affective Neuroscience* 7, no. 2 (2012): 145–59.

Small, G. W., and L. F. Jarvik. "The dementia syndrome." *Lancet* 2, no. 8313 (1982): 1443–6.

Gage, F. H. "Neurogenesis in the adult brain." *Journal of Neuroscience* 22, no. 3 (2002): 612–13.

Small, G. W., et al. "Effects of a 14-day healthy longevity lifestyle program on cognition and brain function." *American Journal of Geriatric Psychiatry* 14, no. 6 (2006): 538–45.

Miller, K. J., et al. "The Memory Fitness Program: cognitive effects of a healthy aging intervention." *American Journal of Geriatric Psychiatry* 20, no. 6 (2012): 514–23.

Small, G. W., et al. "Your brain on Google: patterns of cerebral activation during Internet searching." *American Journal of Geriatric Psychiatry* 17, no. 2 (2009): 116–26.

Ritchie, K. "Mental status examination of an exceptional case of longevity: J. C. aged 118 years." *British Journal of Psychiatry* 166, no. 2 (1995): 229–35.

Whitney, C. R. "Jeanne Calment, world's elder, dies at 122." *New York Times,* Aug 5, 1997. http://www.nytimes.com/1997/08/05/world/jeanne-calment-world-s-elder-dies-at-122.html

Chapter 2:
Mastering Memory

Parker, E. S., et al. "A case of unusual autobiographical remembering." *Neurocase* 12, no. 1 (2006): 35–49.

MacKay, D. G., and L. W. Johnson. "Errors, error detection, error correction and hippocampal-region damage: data and theories." *Neuropsychologica* 51, no. 13 (2013): 2633–50.

Smith, C. N., and Squire, L. R. "Medial temporal lobe activity during retrieval of semantic memory is related to the age of the memory." *Journal of Neuroscience* 29, no. 4 (2009): 9308.

Salthouse T. A., and A. R. Mandell. "Do age-related increases in tip-of-the-tongue experiences signify episodic memory impairments?" *Psychological Science* 24, no. 12 (2013): 2489–97.

Small, G. W., et al. "Effects of a 14-day healthy longevity lifestyle program on cognition and brain function." *American Journal of Geriatric Psychiatry* 14 (2006): 538–45.

Miller, K. J., et al. "The Memory Fitness Program: cognitive effects of a healthy aging intervention." *American Journal of Geriatric Psychiatry* 20, no. 6 (2012): 514–23.

Willis, S. L., et al. "Long-term effects of cognitive training on everyday functional outcomes in older adults. *JAMA* 296, no. 23 (2006): 2805–14.

Rebok, G. W., et al. "Ten-year effects of the advanced cognitive training for independent and vital elderly cognitive training trial on cognition and everyday functioning in older adults." *Journal of the American Geriatrics Society* 62, no. 1 (2014): 16–24.

Chapter 3:
Cut Stress to Sharpen Your Mind

Thoits, P. A. "Stress and health: Major findings and policy implications." *Journal of Health and Social Behavior* 51 (2010): S41–53.

van Ast, V. A., et al. "Modulatory mechanisms of cortisol effects on emotional learning and memory: novel perspectives." *Psychoneuroendocrinology* 38, no. 9 (2013): 1874–82.

Het, S., et al. "A meta-analytic review of the effects of acute cortisol administration on human memory." *Psychoneuroendocrinology* 30, no. 8 (2005): 771–84.

Buchanan, T. W., and W. R. Lovallo. "Enhanced memory for emotional material following stress-level cortisol treatment in humans." *Psychoneuroendocrinology* 26, no. 3 (2001): 307–17.

Ohara, T., et al. "Glucose tolerance status and risk of dementia in the community: the Hisayama study." *Neurology* 77, no. 12 (2011):1126–34.

Johansson, L., et al. "Midlife psychological stress and risk of dementia: a 35-year longitudinal population study." *Brain* 133, pt. 8 (2010): 2217–24.

Johansson, L., et al. "Midlife psychological distress associated with late-life brain atrophy and white matter lesions: a 32-year population study of women." *Psychosomatic Medicine* 74, no. 2 (2012): 120–5.

Johansson, L., et al. "Common psychosocial stressors in middle-aged women related to longstanding distress and increased risk of Alzheimer's disease: a 38-year longitudinal population study." *BMJ Open* 3, no. 9 (2010): e003142. doi: 10.1136/bmjopen-2013-003142.

Norton, M. C., et al. "Early parental death and remarriage of widowed parents as risk factors for Alzheimer disease: the Cache County study." *American Journal of Geriatric Psychiatry* 19, no. 9 (2011): 814–24.

Yehuda, R., et al. "Relationship between cortisol and age-related memory impairments in Holocaust survivors with PTSD." *Psychoneuroendocrinology* 30, no. 7 (2005): 678–87.

Zoladz, P., et al. "Current status on behavioral and biological markers of PTSD: a search for clarity in a conflicting literature." *Neuroscience & Biobehavioral Reviews* 37, no. 5 (2013): 860–95.

Samuelson, K. W. "Post-traumatic stress disorder and declarative memory functioning: a review." *Dialogues in Clinical Neuroscience* 13, no.3 (2011): 346-351.

Cohen, B. E., et al. "Posttraumatic stress disorder and cognitive function: findings from the Mind Your Heart study." *Journal of Clinical Psychiatry* 74, no. 11 (2013): 1063–70.

Thase, M. E. "Comparative effectiveness of psychodynamic psychotherapy and cognitive- behavioral therapy: it's about time, and what's next?" *American Journal of Psychiatry* 170, no. 9 (2013): 953–5.

McGrath, C. L., et al. "Toward a neuroimaging treatment selection biomarker for major depressive disorder." *JAMA Psychiatry* 70, no. 8 (2013): 821–9.

Jorm, A. F. "History of depression as a risk factor for dementia: an updated review." *Australia and New Zealand Journal of Psychiatry* 35, no. 6 (2001): 776–81.

Richard, E., et al. "Late-life depression, mild cognitive impairment, and dementia." *JAMA Neurology* 70, no. 3 (2013): 374–82.

Kumar, A., et al. "Protein binding in patients with late-life depression." *Archives of General Psychiatry* 68, no. 11 (2011): 1143–50.

Lambiase, M. J., et al. "Prospective study of anxiety and incident stroke." *Stroke* 45, no. 2 (2014): 438–4.

Apkarian, A. V., et al. "Brain white matter structural properties predict transition to chronic pain." *Pain* 154, no. 10 (2013): 2160–8.

Apkarian, A. V., et al. "Predicting transition to chronic pain." *Current Opinion in Neurology* 26, no. 4 (2012): 360–7.

Seminowicz, D. A., et al. "Cognitive-behavioral therapy increases prefrontal cortex gray matter in patients with chronic pain." *Journal of Pain* 14, no. 12 (2013): 1573–84.

Morin, C. M., et al. "Monthly fluctuations of insomnia symptoms in a population-based sample." *Sleep* 37, no. 2 (2014): 319–26.

Stickgold, R. "Sleep-dependent memory consolidation." *Nature* 437, no. 7063 (2005): 1272–8.

Benedict, C., et al. "Acute sleep deprivation increases serum levels of neuron-specific enolase (NSE) and S100 calcium binding protein B (S-100B) in healthy young men." *Sleep* 37, no. 1 (2014): 195–8.

Spira, A. P., et al. "Self-reported sleep and β-amyloid deposition in community-dwelling older adults." *JAMA Neurology* 70, no. 12 (2013): 1537–43.

Simpson, N., and D. F. Dinges. "Sleep and inflammation." *Nutrition Reviews* 65, no. 12, pt. 2 (2007): S244–52.

Troxel, W. M., et al. "Sleep symptoms predict the development of the metabolic syndrome." *Sleep* 33, no. 12 (2010): 1633–40.

Xie, L., et al. "Sleep drives metabolite clearance from the adult brain." *Science* 342, no. 6156 (2013): 373–7.

Manber, R., et al. "Cognitive behavioral therapy for insomnia enhances depression outcome in patients with comorbid major depressive disorder and insomnia." *Sleep* 31, no. 4 (2008): 489–95.

Chen, S. T., et al. "Psychological well-being and regional brain amyloid and tau in mild cognitive impairment." *American Journal of Geriatric Psychiatry* 22, no. 4 (2014): 362–9.

Goyal, M., et al. "Meditation programs for psychological stress and well-being: a systematic review and meta-analysis." *JAMA Internal Medicine* 174, no. 3 (2014): 357–68.

Wells, R. E., et al. "Meditation's impact on default mode network and hippocampus in mild cognitive impairment: a pilot study." *Neuroscience Letters* 556 (2013): 15–9.

Vøllestad, J., et al. "Mindfulness- and acceptance-based interventions for anxiety disorders: a systematic review and meta-analysis." *British Journal of Clinical Psychology* 51, no. 3 (2012): 239–60.

Cramer, H., et al. "A systematic review and meta-analysis of yoga for low back pain." *Clinical Journal of Pain* 29, no. 5 (2013): 450–60.

Bhargav, H., et al. "Enhancement of cancer stem cell susceptibility to conventional treatments through complementary yoga therapy: possible cellular and molecular mechanisms." *Journal of Stem Cells* 7, no. 4 (2012): 261–7.

Carek, P., et al. "Exercise for the treatment of depression and anxiety." *International Journal of Psychiatry in Medicine* 41, no. 1 (2011): 15–28.

Wang, Z., et al. "Effect of acupuncture in mild cognitive impairment and Alzheimer's disease: a functional MRI study." *PLoS One* 7, no. 8 (2012): e91160. doi: 10.1371/journal.pone.0042730.

Rubinstein, J. S., et al. "Executive control of cognitive processes in task switching." *Journal of Expermental Psychology: Human Perception and Performance* 27 (2001): 763-97.

Stone, L. "Continuous partial attention." http://lindastone.net/qa/continuous-partial-attention/.

Neuhoff, C. C., and C. Schaefer. "Effects of laughing, smiling, and howling on mood." *Psychological Reports* 91, no. 3, pt. 2 (2002): 1079-80.

Goldin, P. R., et al. "The neural bases of amusement and sadness: a comparison of block contrast and subject-specific emotion intensity regression approaches." *NeuroImage* 27, no. 1 (2005): 26-36.

Kross, E., et al. "Self-talk as a regulatory mechanism: how you do it matters." *Journal of Personality and Social Psychology* 106, no. 2 (2014):304-24.

Muroff, J., et al. "Cognitive behavior therapy for hoarding disorder: follow-up findings and predictors of outcome." *Depression and Anxiety* 31, no. 12 (December 2014): 964–71. doi: 10.1002/da.22222 (November 26, 2013, ePub ahead of print).

Vickers, A. J., et al. "Acupuncture for chronic pain: individual patient data meta-analysis." *Archives of Internal Medicine* 172, no. 19 (2012):1444–53.

Wang, Z., et al. "Acupuncture modulates resting state hippocampal functional connectivity in Alzheimer's disease." *PLoS One* 9, no. 3 (2014): 91160. doi: 10.1371/journal.pone.0091160.

Bangen, K. J., et al. "Brains of optimistic older adults respond less to fearful faces." *Journal of Neuropsychiatry & Clinical Neurosciences* 26, no. 2 (2014): 155-63.

Carney, D. R., et al. "Power posing: brief nonverbal displays affect neuroendocrine levels and risk tolerance." *Psychological Science* 21, no. 10 (October 2010)" 1363–8. doi: 10.1177/0956797610383437 (September 20, 2010, ePub ahead of print).

Ybarra, O., et al. "Mental exercising through simple socializing: social interaction promotes general cognitive functioning." *Personality and Social Psychology Bulletin* 34, no. 2 (2008): 248–59.

Slavich, G. M., et al. "Neural sensitivity to social rejection is associated with inflammatory responses to social stress." *Proceedings of the National Academy of Sciences of the United States of America* 107, no. 33 (2010): 14817–22.

Fox, A. S., et al. "Calling for help is independently modulated by brain systems underlying goal-directed behavior and threat perception." *Proceedings of the National Academy of Sciences of the United States of America* 102, no. 11 (2005): 4176–9.

Chapter 4:
Get Smart with Brain Games

Imtiaz B, et al. "Future directions in Alzheimer's disease from risk factors to prevention." *Biochemical Pharmacology* 88, no. 4 (April 15, 2014): 661–70. doi: 10.1016/j.bcp.2014.01.003 (January 10, 2014, ePub ahead of print).

Gage, F. H. "Neurogenesis in the adult brain." Journal *Neuroscience* 22, no. 3 (2012): 612–3.

Lingineni, R. K., et al. "Factors associated with attention deficit/hyperactivity disorder among US children: results from a national survey." *BMC Pediatrics* 12 (2012): 50. doi: 10.1186/1471-2431-12-50.

Kaplan, J. S., "The effects of shared environment on adult intelligence: a critical review of adoption, twin, and MZA studies." *Developmental Psychology* 48, no. 5 (2012): 1292–8.

Mortensen, E. L., et al. "The association between duration of breastfeeding and adult intelligence." *JAMA* 287, no. 18 (2002): 2365–71.

Schellenberg, E. G. "Music lessons enhance IQ." *Psychological Science* 15, no. 8 (2004): 511–4.

Jaeggi, S. M., et al. "Short- and long-term benefits of cognitive training." *Proceedings of the National Academy of Sciences of the United States of America* 108, no. 25 (2011):10081–6.

Bergman, N.S., et al. "Gains in fluid intelligence after training non-verbal reasoning in 4- year-old children: a controlled, randomized study." *Developmental Science* 14, no. 3 (2011): 591–601.

Borella, E., et al. "Working memory training in old age: an examination of transfer and maintenance effects." *Archives of Clinical Neuropsychology* 28, no. 4 (2013): 331–47.

Hobson, J. A., and A. B. Scheibel. "The brainstem core: sensorimotor integration and behavioral state control." *Neurosciences Research Program Bulletin* 18, no. 1 (1980): 1–173.

Bookheimer, S. Y., et al. "Patterns of brain activation in people at risk for Alzheimer's disease." *New England Journal of Medicine* 343, no. 7 (2000): 450–6.

Luders, E., et al. "Positive correlations between corpus callosum thickness and intelligence." *NeuroImage* 37, no. 4 (2007): 1457–64.

Men, W., et al. "The corpus callosum of Albert Einstein's brain: another clue to his high intelligence?" *Brain* 137, pt. 4 (April 2014): e268. doi:10.1093/brain/awt252 (September 24, 2014, ePub ahead of print).

Maguire, E. A., et al. "Navigation around London by a taxi driver with bilateral hippocampal lesions." *Brain* 129, pt. 11 (2006): 2894–907.

Nutley, S. B., et at. "Music practice is associated with development of working memory during childhood and adolescence."*Frontiers in Human Neuroscience* 7 (2014): 926. doi: 10.3389/fnhum.2013.00926.

Martensson, J., et al. "Growth of language-related brain areas after foreign language learning." NeuroImage. 63, no. 1 (2012): 240–4.

Craik, F. I., et al. "Delaying the onset of Alzheimer disease: bilingualism as a form of cognitive reserve." *Neurology* 75, no. 19 (2010): 1726–9.

Small, G. W., et al. "Your brain on Google: patterns of cerebral activation during Internet searching." *American Journal of Geriatric Psychiatry* 17, no. 2 (2009): 116–26.

Moody, T. D., et al. "Neural activity patterns in older adults following Internet training." *Society for Neuroscience* Meeting, 2009.

Miller, K. J., et al. "Effect of a computerized brain exercise program on cognitive performance in older adults." *American Journal of Geriatric Psychiatry* 21, no. 7 (2003): 655–63.

Rubinstein, J. S., et al. "Executive control of cognitive processes in task switching." *Journal of Expermental Psychology: Human Perception and Performance* 27, no. 4 (2001): 763–97.

Anguera, J. A., et al. "Video game training enhances cognitive control in older adults." *Nature* 501, no. 7465 (2013): 97–101.

Chapter 5:
Food for Thought

Cendri, A., et al. "Cognitive regulation during decision making shifts behavioral control between ventromedial and dorsolateral prefrontal value systems." *Journal of Neuroscience* 32, no. 39 (2012): 13543–4.

Hare, A., et al. "Self-control in decision-making involves modulation of the vmPFC valuation system." *Science* 324, no. 5927 (2009): 646–8.

World Health Organization. "Obesity and overweight." 2003. http://www.who.int/dietphysicalactivity/media/en/gsfs_obesity.pdf.

Hassing, L. B., et al. "Overweight in midlife and risk of dementia: a 40-year follow-up study." *International Journal of Obesity* 33, no. 8 (2009): 893–8.

Raffaitin, C., et al. "Metabolic syndrome and risk for incident Alzheimer's disease or vascular dementia: the Three-City Study." *Diabetes Care* 32, no. 1 (2009): 169–74.

Debette S., et al. "Visceral fat is associated with lower brain volume in healthy middle-aged adults." *Annals of Neurology* 68, no. 2 (2010):136–44.

Cournot, M., et al. "Relation between body mass index and cognitive function in healthy middle-aged men and women." *Neurology* 67, no. 7 (2006): 1208–14.

Gunstad, J., et al. "Improved memory function 12 weeks after bariatric surgery." *Surgery for Obesity and Related Diseases* 7, no. 4 (2011): 465–72.

Barger, J. L., et al. "The retardation of aging by caloric restriction: its significance in the transgenic era." *Experimental Gerontology* 38, no. 11–12 (2003):1343–51.

Fitzpatrick, A. L., et al. "Midlife and late-life obesity and the risk of dementia: cardiovascular health study." *Archives of Neurology* 66, no. 3 (2009): 336–42.

Gillette-Guyonnet, S., et al. "IANA (International Academy on Nutrition and Aging) Expert Group: weight loss and Alzheimer's disease." *Journal of Nutrition, Health, and Aging* 11, no. 1 (2007): 38–48.

Tadahiro, S., et al. "Suppression of oxidative stress by β-hydroxybutyrate, an endogenous histone deacetylase inhibitor." *Science* 339, no. 6116 (2003): 211–4.

World Health Organization. "Global strategy on diet, physical activity, and health." 2006. http://apps.who.int/gb/ebwha/pdf_files/WHA59-REC3/WHA59_REC3-en.pdf.

Small, G. W., et al. "Healthy behavior and memory self-reports in young, middle-aged and older adults." *International Psychogeriatrics* 25, no. 6 (2013): 981–9.

Tamers, S. L., et al. "US and France adult fruit and vegetable consumption patterns: an international comparison." *European Journal of Clinical Nutrition* 63, no. 1 (2009): 11–17.

Sabzghabaee, A. M., et al. "Fruit and vegetable consumption among community dwelling elderly in an Iranian population." *International Journal of Preventive Medicine* 1, no. 2 (2010): 98–102.

Barberger-Gateau, P., et al. "Dietary patterns and risk of dementia: the Three-City cohort study." *Neurology* 69, no. 20 (2007): 1921–30.

Kuhad, A., et al. "Lycopene attenuates diabetes-associated cognitive decline in rats." *Life Sciences* 83, no. 3–4 (2008): 128–34.

Li, Y., et al. "Recent progress on nutraceutical research in prostate cancer." *Cancer and Metastasis Reviews* 33, no. 2–3, (September 2014): 629–40. doi: 10.1007/s10555-013-9478-9 (December 28, 2013, ePub ahead of print).

Akbaraly, T. N., et al. "Chronic inflammation as a determinant of future aging phenotypes." *Canadian Medical Association Journal* 185, no. 16 (2013): E763–70.

Meraz-Ríos, M. A., et al. "Inflammatory process in Alzheimer's disease." *Frontiers in Integrative Neuroscience* 7 (2013): 59. doi: 10.3389/fnint.2013.00059.

Rosenblat, J. D., et al. "Inflamed moods: a review of the interactions between inflammation and mood disorders." *Progress in Neuro-Psychopharmacol & Biological Psychiatry* 53 (August 4, 2014): 23–34. doi: 10.1016/j. pnpbp.2014.01.013. (January 25, 2014; ePub ahead of print).

Horrocks, L. A., and Y. K. Yeo. "Health benefits of docosahexaenoic acid (DHA)." *Pharmacological Research* 40, no. 3 (1999): 211–25.

Muldoom, M. F., et al. "Serum phospholipid docosahexaenonic acid is associated with cognitive functioning during middle adulthood." *Journal of Nutrition* 140, no. 4 (2010): 848–53.

Gardener, H., et al. "Mediterranean diet and white matter hyperintensity volume in the Northern Manhattan Study." *Archives of Neurology* 69, no. 2 (2012): 251–6.

Scarmeas N, et al. "Mediterranean Diet and mild cognitive impairment." *Archives of Neurology* 66, no. 2 (2009): 216–25.

Kien, C. L., et al. "Substituting dietary monounsaturated fat for saturated fat is associated with increased daily physical activity and resting energy expenditure and with changes in mood." *American Journal of Clinical Nutrition* 97, no. 4 (2013): 689–97.

Wansink, B., and L. R. Linder. "Interactions between forms of fat consumption and restaurant bread consumption." *International Journal of Obesity and Related Metabolic Disorders* 27, no. 7 (2003): 866–8.

Martinez-Gonzalez, M. A., et al. "Yogurt consumption, weight gain, and the risk of overweight/obesity: the SUN cohort study." *Nutrition, Metabolism & Cardiovascular Diseases* 24, no. 11 (November 2014): 1189–96. doi: 10.1016/j.numecd.05.015.2014 (June 15, 2014, ePub ahead of print).

Meyer, K. A., et al. "Carbohydrates, dietary fiber, and incident type 2 diabetes in older women." American *Journal of Clinical Nutrition* 71, no. 4 (2000): 921–30.

Wolever, T. M. "Dietary carbohydrates and insulin action in humans." *British Journal of Nutrition* 83, suppl. 1 (2000): S97–102.

Mohan, V., et al. "Effect of brown rice, white rice, and brown rice with legumes on blood glucose and insulin responses in overweight Asian Indians: a randomized controlled trial." *Diabetes Technology & Therapeutics* 16, no. 5 (May 2014): 317–25. doi: 10.1089/dia.2013.0259 (January 21, 2014; ePub ahead of print).

Muñoz-Pareja, M., et al. "Obesity-related eating behaviors are associated with higher food energy density and higher consumption of sugary and alcoholic beverages: a cross-sectional study. *PLoS One* 8, no. 10 (2013): e77137. doi: 10.1371/journal.pone.0077137

Cabrera Escobar, M. A., et al. "Evidence that a tax on sugar sweetened beverages reduces the obesity rate: a meta-analysis." *BMC Public Health* 13 (2013): 1072. doi: 10.1186/1471-2458-13-1072.

Schroeder, J. A., et al. "Nucleus accumbens C-Fos expression is correlated with conditioned place preference to cocaine, morphine and high fat/sugar food consumption." Society for Neuroscience Annual Meeting, 2013. http://www.sfn.org/annual-meeting/neuroscience-2013/abstracts-and-sessions.

Eskelinen M, H., and M. Kivipelto. "Caffeine as a protective factor in dementia and Alzheimer's disease." *Journal of Alzheimer's Disease* 20, suppl. 1 (2010): S167-74.

Qi, H., and S. Li. "Dose-response meta-analysis on coffee, tea and caffeine consumption with risk of Parkinson's disease." *Geriatric & Gerontology International* 14, no. 2 (April 2014): 430–9. doi: 10.1111/ggi.12123 (July 23, 2013, ePub ahead of print).

Chen, X., et al. "Caffeine protects against disruptions of the blood-brain barrier in animal models of Alzheimer's and Parkinson's diseases." *Journal of Alzheimer's Disease* 20, suppl. 1 (2010): S127-41.

Cao, C., et al. "High blood caffeine levels in MCI linked to lack of progression to dementia." *Journal of Alzheimer's Disease* 30, no. 3 (2012): 559–72.

Borota, D., et al. "Post-study caffeine administration enhances memory consolidation in Humans." *Nature Neuroscience* 17, no. 2 (2014): 201–3.

Anstey, K. J., et al. "Alcohol consumption as a risk factor for dementia and cognitive decline: meta-analysis of prospective studies." *American Journal of Geriatric Psychiatry* 17, no. 7 (2009): 542–55.

Wang, J., et al. "Moderate consumption of Cabernet Sauvignon attenuates Abeta neuropathology in a mouse model of Alzheimer's disease." *FASEB Journal* 20, no. 13 (2006): 2313–20.

Liu, D., et al. "Resveratrol prevents impaired cognition induced by chronic unpredictable mild stress in rats." *Progress in Neuro-Psychopharmacology & Biological Psychiatry* 49 (2014): 21–9.

Chapter 6:
Keep Fit for a Younger Brain

Bherer, L., et al. "A review of the effects of physical activity and exercise on cognitive and brain functions in older adults." *Journal of Aging Research* 2013: Article ID 657508. http://www.hindawi.com/journals/jar/2013/657508/#B52.

Kramer, A. F., et al. "Environmental influences on cognitive and brain plasticity during aging." *Journals of Gerontology* 59, no. 9 (2004): 940–57.

Weinstein, G., et al. "Serum brain-derived neurotrophic factor and the risk for dementia: the Framingham Heart Study." *JAMA Neurology* 71, no. 1 (2014): 55–61. doi: 10.1001/jamaneurol.2013.4781.

Carek, P., et al. "Exercise for the treatment of depression and anxiety." *International Journal of Psychiatry in Medicine* 41, no. 1 (2011): 15–28.

Yaffe, K., et al. *Alzheimer's Association International Conference*, 2013. Boston, MA.

Defina LF, et al. "Middle-aged people who take up exercise: The association between midlife cardiorespiratory fitness levels and later-life dementia: a cohort study." *Annals of Internal Medicine* 158, no. 3 (2013): 162–8.

Bullain, S. S., et al. "Poor physical performance and dementia in the oldest old: the 90+ study." *JAMA Neurology* 70, no. 1 (2013): 107–13.

Erickson, K. I., et al. "Aerobic fitness is associated with hippocampal volume in elderly humans." *Hippocampus* 19, no. 10 (2009): 1030–9.

Killgore, W. D., et al. "Physical exercise habits correlate with gray matter volume of the hippocampus in healthy adult humans." *Scientific Reports* 3, no. 3475 (2013). doi: 10.1038/srep03457.

Erickson, K. I., et al. "Exercise training increases size of hippocampus and improves memory." *Proceedings of the National Academy of Sciences of the United States of America* 108, no. 7 (2010): 3017–22.

Jeon, C. Y., et al. "Physical activity of moderate intensity and risk of type 2 diabetes: a systematic review." *Diabetes Care* 30, no. 3 (2007): 744–52.

Ohara, T., et al. "Glucose tolerance status and risk of dementia in the community: the Hisayama study." *Neurology* 77, no. 12 (2011): 1126–34.

Allison, D. B., et al. "Annual deaths attributed to obesity in the United States." *JAMA* 282, no. 16 (1999): 1530–8.

Chodzko-Zajko, W. J., et al. "American College of Sports Medicine position stand: exercise and physical activity for older adults." *Medical Science in Sports & Exercise* 41, no. 7 (2009): 1510–30.

Scarapicchia, T. M. F., et al. "The motivational effects of social contagion on exercise participation in young female adults." *Journal of Sport & Exercise Psychology* 35, no. 6 (2013): 563–75.

Etgen, T., et al. "Physical activity and incident cognitive impairment in elderly persons: the INVADE study." *Archives of Internal Medicine* 170, no. 2 (2010): 1886–93.

Larson, E. B., et al. "Exercise is associated with reduced risk for incident dementia among persons 65 years of and older." *Annals of Internal Medicine* 144, no. 2 (2006): 73–81.

Lang, P. J., et al. "Emotion, motivation, and anxiety: brain mechanisms and psychophysiology." *Biological Psychiatry* 44, no. 12 (1998): 1248–63.

Lally, P., et al. "How are habits formed: modelling habit formation in the real world." *European Journal of Social Psychology* 40, no. 6 (2010): 998–1009.

Sarkisian, C. A., et al. "Pilot test of an attribution retraining intervention to raise walking levels in sedentary older adults." *Journal of American Geriatric Society* 55, no. 11 (2007): 1842–6.

Scheef, L., et al. "An fMRI study on the acute effects of exercise on pain processing in trained athletes." *Pain* 153, no. 8 (2012): 1702–14.

Schoenfeld, T. J., et al. "Physical exercise prevents stress-
induced activation of granule neurons and enhances local
inhibitory mechanisms in the dentate gyrus." *Journal of
Neuroscience* 33, no. 18 (2013): 7770–7.

Faul, M., et al. "Traumatic brain injury in the United States:
emergency department visits, hospitalizations, and deaths."
US department of Health and Human Services, Centers
for Disease Control and Prevention, National Center for
Injury Prevention and Control, 2010. http://www.cdc.gov/
traumaticbraininjury/pdf/blue_book.pdf.

Small, G. W., et al. "PET scanning of brain tau in retired
National Football League players." *American Journal of
Geriatric Psychiatry* 21, no. 2 (2013): 138–44.

Jordan, B. D. "Apolipoprotein E epsilon4 associated with
chronic traumatic brain injury in boxing." *JAMA* 278, no. 2
(1997): 136–40.

Shively S., et al. "Dementia resulting from traumatic brain
injury: what is the pathology?" *Archives of Neurology* 69, no.
10 (2012): 1245–51.

Mielke, M. M., et al. "Head trauma and in vivo measures of
amyloid and neurodegeneration in a population-based
study." *Neurology* 82, no. 1 (2014): 70–6.

Gottlieb, J., et al. "Information-seeking, curiosity, and
attention: computational and neural mechanisms." *Trends in
Cognitive Sciences* 17, no. 11 (2013): 585–93.

Warburton, D. E., et al. "Blood volume expansion and function:
effects of training modality." *Medicine & Science in Sports &
Exercise* 36, no. 6 (2004): 991–1000.

Schmidt, W. D., et al. "Effects of long versus short bout exercise on fitness and weight loss in overweight females." *Journal of the American College of Nutrition.* 20, no. 5 (2001): 494–501.

Jones, A. M., et al. "A 1% treadmill grade most accurately reflects the energetic cost of outdoor running." *Journal of Sports Sciences* 14, no. 4 (1996): 321–7.

Johnson, R. A., and R. L. Meadows. "Dog-walking: motivation for adherence to a walking program." *Clinical Nursing Research* 19, no. 4 (2010): 387–402.

Abou-Dest, A., et al. "Swimming as a positive moderator of cognitive aging: a cross-sectional study with a multitask approach." *Journal of Aging Research* 19 (2012): 387–402.

Pluim, B. M., et al. "Health benefits of tennis." *British Journal of Sports Medicine* 41 (2007): 760–8.

Pilgramm, S., et al. "Differential activation of the lateral premotor cortex during action observation." *BMC Neuroscience* 11 (2010): 89.

Kattenstroth, J. C., et al. "Superior sensory, motor, and cognitive performance in elderly individuals with multi-year dancing activities." *Frontiers in Aging Neuroscience* 2 (2010): 31.

Crum, A. J., and E. J. Langer. "Mind-set matters: exercise and the placebo effect." *Psychological Science* 18, no. 2 (2007): 165–71.

Martinsen, E. W., et al. "Comparing aerobic with nonaerobic forms of exercise in the treatment of clinical depression: a randomized trial." *Comprehensive Psychiatry* 30, no. 4 (1989): 324–31.

Marzolini S, et al. "The effects of an aerobic and resistance exercise training program on cognition following stroke." *Neurorehabilitation & Neural Repair* 27, no. 5. (2013): 392–402.

Caffilhas, R. C., et al. "Spatial memory is improved by aerobic and resistance exercise through divergent molecular mechanisms." *Neuroscience* 202 (2012): 309–17.

Nagamatsu, L. S., et al. "Physical activity improves verbal and spatial memory in older adults with probable mild cognitive impairment: a 6-month randomized controlled trial." *Journal of Aging Research* 2013: Article ID 861893. doi: 10.1155/2013/861893.

Nelson, M. E., et al. "Physical activity and public health in older adults: recommendation   from the American College of Sports Medicine and the American Heart Association." *Medicine & Science in Sports & Exercise* 39, no. 8 (2007): 1435–45.

Verghagen, E., et al. "The effect of a proprioceptive balance board training program for the prevention of ankle sprains: a prospective controlled trial. *American Journal of Sports Medicine* 32, no. 6 (2004): 138593.

Makizako, H., et al. "Poor balance and lower gray matter volume predict falls in older adults with mild cognitive impairment." *BMC Neurology* 13 (2013): 102. doi: 10.1186/1471-2377-13-102.

Delbaere, K., et al. "Mild cognitive impairment as a predictor of falls in community-dwelling older people." *American Journal of Geriatric Psychiatry* 20, no. 10 (2012): 845–53.

Mersmann, F., et al. "Young and old adults prioritize dynamic stability control following gait perturbations when performing a concurrent cognitive task." *Gait & Posture* 37, no. 3 (2013): 373–7.

Hackney, M. E., and S. L. Wolf. "Impact of Tai Chi Chu'an practice on balance and mobility in older adults: an integrative review of 20 years of research." *Journal of*

Geriatric Physical Therapy 37, no. 3 (December 20, 2013): 127–35. doi: 10.1519/JPT.0b013e3182abe784 (July– September, 2014; ePub ahead of print).

Mortimer, J., et al. "Changes in brain volume and cognition in a randomized trial of exercise and social interaction in a community-based sample of non-demented Chinese elders." *Journal of Alzheimer's Disease* 30, no. 4 (2012): 757–66.

Kloubec, J. A. "Pilates for improvement of muscle endurance, flexibility, balance, and posture. *Journal of Strength & Conditioning Research* 24, no. 3 (2010): 661–7.

Sekendiz, B., et al. "Effects of Swiss-ball core strength training on strength, endurance, flexibility, and balance in sedentary women". *Journal of Strength & Conditioning Research* 24, no. 11 (2010): 3032–40.

Hariprasad, V. R., et al. "Yoga increases the volume of the hippocampus in elderly subjects." *Indian Journal of Psychiatry* 55, suppl. 3 (2013): S394-6.

Froeliger, B., et al. "Yoga meditation practitioners exhibit greater gray matter volume and fewer reported cognitive failures: results of a preliminary voxel-based morphometric analysis." *Evidence-Based Complementary and Alternative Medicine* 2012: Article ID 821307. doi: 10.1155/2012/821307.

Chapter 7:
Good Friends Make Happy Neurons

Dufouil, C., et al. "Older age at retirement is associated with decreased risk of dementia." Alzheimer's Association International Conference, 2013. http://www.ilcfrance.org/ actualites/docs/2013/AbstractAAIC2013_CDufouil.pdf.

Sireteanu, R., et al. "Graphical illustration and functional neuroimaging of visual hallucinations during prolonged blindfolding: a comparison to visual imagery." *Perception* 37, no. 12 (2008): 1805–21.

Makinodan, M., et al. "A critical period for social experience–dependent oligodendrocyte maturation and myelination." *Science* 337, no. 6100 (2012): 1357–60.

Coan, J. A., et al. "Lending a hand: social regulation of the neural response to threat." *Psychological Science* 17, no. 12 (2006): 1032–9.

Dalton, K. M., et al. "Gaze-fixation, brain activation, and amygdala volume in unaffected siblings of individuals with autism." *Biological Psychiatry* 61, no. 4 (2007): 512–20.

Nacewicz, B. M., et al. "Amygdala volume and nonverbal social impairment in adolescent and adult males with autism." *Archives of General Psychiatry* 63, no. 12 (2006): 1417–28.

Kross, E., et al. "Social rejection shares somatosensory representations with physical pain." *Proceedings of the National Academy of Sciences of the UnitedStates of America* 108, no. 15 (2011): 6270–5.

Kubzansky, L. D., et al. "Protocol for an experimental investigation of the roles of oxytocin and social support in neuroendocrine, cardiovascular, and subjective responses to stress across age and gender." *BMC Public Health* 9 (2009): 481. doi: 10.1186/1471- 2458-9-481.

Glass, T. A., et al. "Population based study of social and productive activities as predictors of survival among elderly Americans." *British Medical Journal* 319, no. 7208 (1999): 478–83.

Ybarra, O., et al. "Mental exercising through simple socializing: social interaction promotes general cognitive functioning." *Personality and Social Psychology Bulletin* 34, no. 2 (2008): 248–59.

Holwerda, T. J., et al. "Feelings of loneliness, but not social isolation, predict dementia onset: results from the Amsterdam Study of the Elderly (AMSTEL)." *Journal of Neurology, Neurosurgery & Psychiatry* 85, no. 2 (2014):135–42.

McGivern, R. F., et al. "Cognitive efficiency on a match to sample task decreases at the onset of puberty in children." *Brain and Cognition* 50, no. 1 (2002): 73–89.

Blakemore, S. J., and S. Choudhury. "Development of the adolescent brain: implications for executive function and social cognition." *Journal of Child Psychology and Psychiatry* 47, no. 3–4 (2006): 296–312. den Ouden, H. E. M., et al. "Thinking about intentions." *NeuroImage* 28, no. 4 (2005): 787–96.

Carr, L., et al. "Neural mechanisms of empathy in humans: a relay from neural systems for imitation to limbic areas." *Proceedings of the National Academy of Sciences of the UnitedStates of America* 100, no. 9 (2003): 5497–5502.

Singer, T., et al. "Empathy for pain involves the affective but not sensory components of pain." *Science* 303, no. 5661 (2004): 1157–62.

Isen, A. M., et al. "Positive affect facilitates creative problem solving." *Journal of Personality and Social Psychology* 52, no. 6 (1987) 122–31.

Vrticka, P., et al. "The neural basis of humour processing." *Nature Reviews Neuroscience* 14, no. 12 (2013): 860–8.

Samson, A. C., et al. "Cognitive humor processing: different logical mechanisms in nonverbal cartoons — an fMRI study." *Social Neuroscience* 3, no. 2 (2008):125–40.

Bast, E. S., and E. M. Berry. "Laugh away the fat? Therapeutic humor in the control of stress- induced emotional eating." *Rambam Maimonides Medical Journal* 5, no. 1 (2014): e0007. doi: 10.5041/RMMJ.10141.

Toda, M., and H. Ichikawa. "Effect of laughter on salivary flow rates and levels of chromogranin A in young adults and elderly people." *Environmental Health and Preventive Medicine* 17, no. 6 (2012): 494–9.

Leuner, B., et al. "Sexual experience promotes adult neurogenesis in the hippocampus despite an initial elevation in stress hormones." *PLoS One* 5, no. 7 (2010): e11597. doi: 10.1317/journal.pone.0011597.

Smith, G. D., S. Frankel, and J. Yarnell. "Sex and death, are they related? Findings from the Caerphilly cohort study." *British Medical Journal* 315, no. 7123 (1997): 1641–4.

Charnetski, C. J., and F. X. Brennan. "Sexual frequency and salivary immunoglobulin A (IgA)." *Psychological Reports* 94, pt. 1 (2004): 839–44.

Giles, L. C., et al. "Effect of social networks on 10-year survival in very old Australians: the Australian longitudinal study of aging." *Journal of Epidemiology and Community Health* 59, no. 7 (2005): 574–9.

Grewen, K. M., et al. "Warm partner contact is related to lower cardiovascular reactivity." *Journal of Behavioral Medicine* 29, no. 3 (2003): 123–30.

Bakermans-Kranenburg, M. J., and M. H. van IJzendoorn. "A sniff of trust: meta-analysis of the effects of intranasal oxytocin administration on face recognition, trust to in-group, and trust to out-group." *Psychoneuroendocrinology* 37, no. 3 (2012): 438–43.

Chapter 8:
Mind Your Medicine

Singh-Manoux, A., et al. "Timing of onset of cognitive decline: results from Whitehall II prospective cohort study." *British Medical Journal* 344 (2012): d7622.

Sherman, R., and J. Hickner. "Academic physicians use placebos in clinical practice and believe in the mind-body connection. *Journal of General Internal Medicine* 23, no. 1 (2008): 7–10.

Wager, T. D., et al. "Placebo-induced changes in fMRI in the anticipation and experience of pain." *Science* 303, no. 5061 (2004): 1162–7.

Rogers, S. L., et al. "Donepezil improves cognition and global function in Alzheimer's disease: a 15-week, double-blind, placebo-controlled study. Donepizil Study Group" *Archives of Internal Medicine* 158, no. 9 (1998): 1021–31.

Lidstone, S. C., and A. J. Stoessl. "Understanding the placebo effect: contributions from neuroimaging." *Molecular Imaging and Biology* 9, no. 4 (2007): 176–85.

Chin, J. J. "Doctor-patient relationship: from medical paternalism to enhanced autonomy." *Singapore Medical Journal* 43, no. 3 (2002): 152–5.

Pew Research Internet Project: Health Fact Sheet. http://www.pewinternet.org/fact- sheets/health-fact-sheet/.

Small, G. W., and L. F. Jarvik. "The dementia syndrome." *Lancet* 2, no. 8313 (1982): 1443–6.

Bettermann, K., et al. "Statins, risk of dementia, and cognitive function: secondary analysis of the Ginkgo Evaluation of Memory Study." *Journal of Stroke & Cerebrovascular Diseases* 21, no. 6 (2012): 436–44.

McGuinness, B., et al. "Statins for the treatment of dementia." Cochrane Database of Systemic Reviews August 4, 2010; (8):CD007514.

Evans, M. A., and B. A. Golomb. "Statin-associated adverse cognitive effects: survey results from 171 patients." *Pharmacotherapy* 29, no. 7 (2009): 800–11.

Bernick, C., et al. "Statins and cognitive function in the elderly: the Cardiovascular Health Study." *Neurology* 65, no. 9 (2005): 1388–94.

Wong, W. B., et al. "Statins in the prevention of dementia and Alzheimer's disease: a meta- analysis of observational studies and an assessment of confounding." *Pharmacoepidemiol Drug Safety* 22, no. 4 (2013): 345–58.

Hasnain, M., et al. "Possible role of vascular risk factors in Alzheimer's disease and vascular dementia." *Current Pharmaceutical Design* 20, no. 38 (2014); 6007–13.

Braskie, M. N., et al. "Vascular health risks and fMRI activation during a memory task in older adults." *Neurobiology of Aging* 31, no. 9 (2010): 1532–42.

Waldstein, S. R., et al. "Nonsteroidal anti-inflammatory drugs, aspirin, and cognitive function in the Baltimore longitudinal study of aging." *Journal of the American Geriatrics Society* 58, no. 1 (2010): 38–43.

Breitner, J. C., et al. "Extended results of the Alzheimer's disease anti-inflammatory prevention trial." *Alzheimer's & Dementia* 7, no. 4 (2011): 402–11.

Schilling, A., et al. "Acetaminophen: old drug, new warnings." *Cleveland Clinic Journal of Medicine* 77, no. 1 (2010): 19–27.

Trumic, E., et al. "Prevalence of polypharmacy and drug interaction among hospitalized patients: opportunities and responsibilities in pharmaceutical care." Materia Socio Med*ica* 24, no. 2 (2012): 68–72.

Small, G. W., "Alzheimer's disease and other dementing disorders." In the *Comprehensive Textbook of Psychiatry, 9th Edition,* edited by B. J., and V. A. Sadock, 4058–65. Baltimore: Williams & Wilkins, 2009.

Silverman, D. H. S., et al. "Long-term effects of donepezil versus placebo on regional brain metabolism in minimally impaired subjects." Alzheimer's Association, 2008 International Conference on Alzheimer's Disease (ICAD).

Petersen, R. C., et al. "Vitamin E and donepezil for the treatment of mild cognitive impairment." *New England Journal of Medicine* 352, no. 23 (2005): 2379–88.

Snowball, A., et al. "Long-term enhancement of brain function and cognition using cognitive training and brain stimulation." *Current Biology* 23, no. 11 (2013): 987–92.

Martin, D. M., et al. "Can transcranial direct current stimulation enhance outcomes from cognitive training? A randomized controlled trial in healthy participants." *International Journal of Neuropsychopharmacology* 16 (2013):1927–36.

Sripada, R. K., et al. "DHEA enhances emotion regulation neurocircuits and modulates memory for emotional stimuli." *International Journal of Neuropsychopharmacology* 38, no. 9 (2013): 1798–807.

Alhaj, H. A., et al. "Effect of DHEA administration on episodic memory, cortisol, and mood in healthy young men: a double-blind, placebo-controlled study." *Psychopharmacologia* 188, no. 4 (2006): 541–51.

Baker, L. D., et al. "Effects of growth hormone-releasing hormone on cognitive function in adults with mild cognitive impairment and healthy older adults: results of a controlled trial." *Archives of Neurology* 69, no. 11 (2012): 1420–9.

Nelson, H. D., et al. "Menopausal hormone therapy for the primary prevention of chronic conditions: a systematic review to update the US Preventive Services Task Force recommendations." *Annals of Internal Medicine* 157, no. 2 (2012):104–13.

Maki, P. M. "Critical window hypothesis of hormone therapy and cognition: a scientific update on clinical studies." *Menopause* 20, no. 6 (2013): 695–709.

Maki, P. M. "Minireview: effects of different HT formulations on cognition." *Endocrinology* 153, no. 8 (2012): 3564–70.

Holland J., et al. "Testosterone levels and cognition in elderly men: a review." *Maturitas* 69, no. 4 (2011):322–37.

Maki, P. M., et al. "Intramuscular testosterone treatment in elderly men: evidence of memory decline and altered brain function." *Journal of Clinical Endocrinology & Metabolism* 92, no. 11 (2007): 4107–14.

Davison, S. L., et al. "Testosterone improves verbal learning and memory in postmenopausal women: results from a pilot study." *Maturitas* 70, no. 3 (2011): 307–11.

Dickinson, A., and D. MacKay. "Health habits and other characteristics of dietary supplement users: a review." *Nutrition Journal* February 6, 2013. doi: 10.1186/1475-2891-13-14.

Fortmann, S. P., et al. "Vitamin, mineral, and multivitamin supplements for the primary prevention of cardiovascular disease and cancer: A systematic evidence review for the US Preventive Services Task Force." *Annals of Internal Medicine* 159, no. 12 (2013): 824–834. doi: 10.7326/0003-4819-159-12-201312170-00729.

Guallar, E., et al. "Enough is enough: stop wasting money on vitamin and mineral supplements." *Annals of Internal Medicine* 159, no. 12 (2013): 850–1.

Dysken, M. W., et al. "Effect of vitamin E and memantine on functional decline in Alzheimer's disease: the TEAM-AD VA cooperative randomized trial." *JAMA* 311, no. 1 (2014): 33–44.

Kang, J. H., et al. "Vitamin E, vitamin C, beta carotene, and cognitive function among women with or at risk of cardiovascular disease: the Women's Antioxidant and Cardiovascular Study." *Circulation* 119, no. 21 (2009): 2749–51.

Bookheimer, S. Y., et al. "Pomegranate juice augments memory and fMRI activity in middle- aged and older adults with mild memory complaints." Evidence-Base Complementary and Alternative Med*icine* 2013: Article ID 946298. doi: 10.1155/2013/946298.

Riggs, K. M., et al. "Relations of vitamin B-12, vitamin B-6, folate, and homocysteine to cognitive performance in the Normative Aging Study." *American Journal of Clinical Nutrition* 63, no. 3 (1996): 306–14.

Moore, E. M., et al. "Among vitamin B12 deficient older people, high folate levels are associated with worse cognitive function: combined data from three cohorts." *Journal of Alzheimer's Disease* 39, no. 3 (2014): 661–8.

Smith, A. D., et al. "Homocysteine-lowering by B vitamins slows the rate of accelerated brain atrophy in mild cognitive impairment: a randomized controlled trial." *PLoS One* 5, no. 9 (2010): e12244.

Politis, A., et al. "Vitamin B12 levels in Alzheimer's disease: association with clinical features and cytokine production." *Journal of Alzheimer's Disease* 19, no. 2 (2010): 481–8.

Llewellyn, D. J., et al. "Vitamin D and risk of cognitive decline in elderly persons." *Archives of Internal Medicine* 170, no. 13 (2010): 1135–41.

Annewiler, C., et al. "Dietary intake of vitamin D and cognition in older women: a large population-based study." *Neurology* 75, no. 20 (2010): 1810–6.

Rossom, R. C., et al. "Calcium and vitamin D supplementation and cognitive impairment in the women's health initiative." *Journal of the American Geriatric Society* 60, no. 12 (2012):2197–205.

Rocha Araujo, D. M., et al. "What is the effectiveness of the use of polyunsaturated fatty acid omega-3 in the treatment of depression?" *Expert Review of Neurotherapeutics* 10, no. 7 (2010): 1117–29.

Witte, A. V., et al. "Long-chain omega-3 fatty acids improve brain function and structure in older adults." *Cerebral Cortex* 24, no. 11 (November 2014): 3059–68. doi: 10.1093/cercor/bht163. (June 24, 2013, ePub ahead of print.)

Pottala, J. V., et al. "Higher RBC EPA + DHA corresponds with larger total brain and hippocampal volumes: WHIMS-MRI Study." *Neurology* 82, no. 5 (2014): 435–42. Alzheimer's Disease International. "Prevalence of dementia worldwide." http://www.alz.co.uk/adi/pdf/prevalence.pdf.

Ringman, J. M., et al. "Oral curcumin for Alzheimer's disease: tolerability and efficacy in a 24-week randomized, double blind, placebo-controlled study." *Alzheimer's Research & Therapy* 4, no. 5 (2012): 43.

Snitz, B. E., et al. "Ginkgo biloba for preventing cognitive decline in older adults: a randomized trial." *JAMA* 302, no. 24 (2009): 2663–70.

Rafii, M. S., et al. "A phase II trial of huperzine A in mild to moderate Alzheimer disease." *Neurology* 76, no. 16 (2011): 1389–94.

Sun, Q. Q., et al. "Huperzine-A capsules enhance memory and learning performance in 34 pairs of matched adolescent students." *Zhongguo Yao Li Xue Bao* 20, no. 7 (1999): 601–3.

Vakhapova, V., et al. "Phosphatidylserine containing omega-3 fatty acids may improve memory abilities in non-demented elderly with memory complaints: a double-blind placebo-controlled trial." *Dementia and Geriatric Cognitive Disorders* 29, no. 5 (2010): 467–74.

Jorissen, B. L., et al. "The influence of soy-derived phosphatidylserine on cognition in age- associated memory impairment." *Nutritional Neuroscience* 4, no. 2 (2001): 121–34.

Crook, T. H., et al. "Effects of phosphatidylserine in age-associated memory impairment. *Neurology.*" 41, no. 5 (1991): 644–9.

Chapter 9:
The 2-Week Younger Brain Program

Pagoto, S., et al. "Initial investigation of behavioral activation therapy for co-morbid major depressive disorder and obesity." *Psychotherapy* 45, no. 3 (2008): 410–5.

Small, G. W., et al. "Effects of a 14-day healthy longevity lifestyle
program on cognition and brain function." *American Journal
of Geriatric Psychiatry* 14, no. 6 (2006): 538–45.

Small, G. W., et al. "Healthy behavior and memory self-reports
in young, middle-aged and older adults." *International
Psychogeriatrics* 25, no. 6 (2013): 981–9.

Chen, S. T., et al. "Modifiable risk factors for Alzheimer disease
and subjective memory impairment across age groups."
PLoS One 9, no. 6 (2014): e98630. doi:10.1371/journal
.pone.0098630.

Miller, K. J., et al. "The Memory Fitness Program: cognitive
effects of a healthy aging intervention." *American Journal of
Geriatric Psychiatry* 20, no. 6 (2012): 514–23.

Knowler, W. C., et al. "Reduction in the incidence of type 2
diabetes with lifestyle intervention or metformin." *New
England Journal of Medicine* 346, no. 6 (2002): 393–403.

Blumenthal, J. A., et al. "Usefulness of psychosocial treatment
of mental stress-induced myocardial ischemia in men."
American Journal of Cardiology 89, no. 2 (2002): 164–8.

Key, T. J., et al. "Health effects of vegetarian and vegan diets."
Proceedings of the Nutrition Society 65, no. 1 (2006): 35–41.

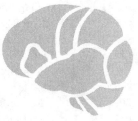

Index

2-Week (14-Day) Younger Brain
Program, ix–x, 3–4, 48, 84, 92, 132,
136, 195–235
    baseline abilities, 202
    building brain synergy, 197–199
    detailed program, 202–233
    feedback, 196–197
    mental exercises, 201. *See also*
        Brain training
    milestones, 196, 218, 233
    physical fitness, 200–201. *See
        also* Physical exercise
    sample meal ideas, 198–199. *See
        also* Diet and nutrition

A
AARP, 239
Acetaminophen (Tylenol), 175–176,
    180

Acetylcholine, 182–183, 192
Acetyl-l-carnitine supplements,
    190
Acupressure, 72
Acupuncture, 71–72
ADHD. *See* Attention deficit
    hyperactivity disorder
Administration for Community
    Living, 239
Adrenal glands, 21–22
Adrenaline, 22, 62
Aerobic fitness, 141–144. *See also*
    Physical exercise
    cycling, 138–139, 142
    dancing, 143
    household chores, 143
    racquet sports, 143
    shopping at the mall, 143–144
    swimming, 142–143

walking for fitness, 141–142. *See also* Walking

Agoraphobia, 62

Ahmanson-Lovelace Brain Mapping Center, 164–165

Alcohol consumption, 124–126
    acetaminophen and, 180
    alcoholism, 110–111, 124, 180
    benefits of moderate consumption, 125–126, 200
    brain damage, 124
    liver and kidney problems and, 180

Aleve (naproxen), 179, 180

Alzheimer Europe, 240

Alzheimer's Association, 240, 241

Alzheimer's disease
    acetylcholine deficiency and, 182–183, 192
    acupuncture and, 72
    amyloid plaques, 13, 61, 126, 178–179
    anti-inflammatory drugs, 179–180
    as cause of dementia, 13, 17
    coconut oil, 119
    delaying retirement to reduce risk of, 151
    docosahexaenoic acid and, 119
    education level and, 18, 78
    genetics and, 16–17, 56, 139
    homocysteine blood levels and risk of, 191
    medications for, 182–183
    menopause and, 186
    mild cognitive impairment and, 183–184
    physical exercise and, 16
    plaques and tangles, 13–14, 183–184, 190
    sleep issues and, 65
    stress and, 58, 22, 155
    tau tangles, 13, 61, 138–139
    vitamin E and, 189

Alzheimer's Disease Education & Referral Center, 240

Alzheimer's Foundation of America, 240

American Academy of Neurology, 240

American Association for Geriatric Psychiatry, 240

American College of Sports Medicine, 146

American Geriatrics Society, 240

American Heart Association, 146

American Psychiatric Association, 110–111, 241

American Psychological Association, 241

American Society on Aging, 241

Amitriptyline (Elavil), 185

Amnesia, 36, 124

Amygdala, 19, 36–37, 53, 61, 138, 154

Anemia, 23, 175

Angina, 168

Animal studies

Ankylosing spondylitis, 166

Anterograde amnesia, 36

Antiaging clinics, 187

Antidepressants, 60–61
    confusion and mood alterations from, 182, 184–185
    effect on memory, 184–185
    effect on pain, 63
    effectiveness compared to exercise, 128
    first vs. second generation, 185
    selective seratonin reuptake inhibitors, 185

Anti-inflammatory drugs, 67, 179–180

Antioxidants, 126, 116–118
    acetyl-l-carnitine, 190
    in alcohol, 126
    coenzyme Q10, 190
    flavonoids, 117

free radicals, 116
fruits and vegetables, 23–24,
    116–117
phytonutrients, 117
polyphenol, 116, 190
resveratrol, 126
supplements, 190
Anxiety, 53–54, 58–59, 62, 67–68,
    72–73, 78, 182
APOE. *See* Apolipoprotein E
Apolipoprotein E (APOE), 16–19
Aricept (donepezil), 173, 182–184
Arthritis, 119, 166, 179–180
Asthma, 21, 62
Atherosclerosis, 177
Atrophy (brain shrinkage), 11, 58, 66
Attention deficit hyperactivity
    disorder (ADHD), 79
Attentive listening, 165
Autism, 154
Autobiographical memory. *See*
    Photographic memory
Axons, 5, 152–153

B
Baby boomers, 3–4, 19–20, 239
    life expectancy, 17, 25
Balance balls and boards, 148–149
Balance training, 147–150. *See also*
    Physical exercise; Tai chi; Yoga
    balance balls and boards, 148–149
    cerebellum and, 14–15, 87
    the flamingo, 147–148, 211
    heel-toe walk, 223
    training program, 147
Bariatric surgery, 114
BDNF. *See* Brain-derived
    neurotrophic factor
Beans, 117, 120, 122, 200
Beta-carotene, 190
Bilingualism, 88–89
Binge-eating disorder, 110–111
Blood clots, 187–188
Blood pressure

controlling, 141, 168, 178–179,
    192. *See also* Physical; Stress
    management
elevated, 24, 54
high (hypertension), 21, 54, 62,
    106, 118, 141, 177–179, 193
metabolic syndrome and, 112
Blood sugar, 112, 155, 122–123, 144,
    185
Blood vessels
    nitric oxide and, 178
    optimal blood flow, 5
    scarring of brain blood vessels,
        58, 121, 177
    substances that dilate, 111, 125.
        See also Blood pressure
    thickening of, 178–179
BMC Public Health, 124
BMI. *See* Body mass index
Body mass index (BMI), 112–113
Bone density, 144
Botox injections, 2
Brain aging, 5–6. *See also*
    Alzheimer's disease; Dementia
    anesthesia and, 3, 23
    atrophy, 11, 58, 66
    causes of, 1–2
    normal, 14
    scarring of brain blood vessels,
        58, 121, 177
    stages of, 13–14
Brain anatomy
    amygdala, 19, 36–37, 53, 61, 138,
        154
    anterior cingulate, 165
    axons, 5, 152–153
    Broca's area, 14–15, 87, 156
    cerebellum, 14–15, 87
    corpus callosum, 11, 87–88
    dendrites, 152–153
    effects of brain training, 24–25
    emotional and reactive centers,
        53, 61
    empathy center, 164–165

executive control and thinking
 centers, 53
food cravings, 107
frontal lobe, 11, 14–15, 36–37,
 86–87, 154–156, 164–165
hippocampus, 14, 36–37, 61,
 88–89, 130, 168, 173
hypothalamus, 154
insula, 61, 155, 164–165
left vs. right sides of, 13, 84–85
myelin, 5, 152–153
neurons, 5–6, 18–19, 84–87
parietal lobe, 14–15, 87
prefrontal cortex, 107, 167
reticular formation, 84
sensorimotor strip, 14–15, 156
somatosensory cortex, 155
spinal cord, 84
synapses, 5, 153
temporal lobe, 14–15, 59, 72,
 87–89, 156, 163
ventromedial cortex, 107
visual cortex, 14–15, 87, 156
white matter, 121, 153
Brain cell death. See Stroke
Brain Den website, 237
Brain health, 1–2. See also 2-Week
 Younger Brain program
 aging and, 5–6. See also Brain
  aging
 diagnosing, 23
 essential functions for a young
  brain, 10
 healthy lifestyle choices and, 4
 mental exercises to improve, 4
 nature vs. nurture, 18
 outward manifestations of,
  11–12
 resources, 239–243
Brain inflammation, 73, 118, 191
Brain shrinkage. See atrophy under
 Brain aging
Brain Teasers website, 237
Brain training, 75–79, 86–88,

92–103, 204
 advanced games, 96–98, 99, 102
 beginner games, 77, 92–94, 99, 100
 Changing Words exercise, 93, 100
 choosing the right exercises, 90–91
 Concentration matching game,
  82–83
 Counting Squares exercise, 93, 100
 cross-training, 84, 135–136
 crossword puzzles, 44, 77, 85, 92,
  204, 211
 Finding Colors, 95, 101
 Finicky Frank, 98, 103
 Hidden Proverb exercise, 95, 102
 Hypothetical Country, 96–97, 102
 increasing difficulty levels, 77–78
 intermediate level games, 77–78,
  94–96, 99, 101
 Jigsaw Brain Breaks, 94, 96, 100,
  101
 jigsaw puzzles, 75, 84, 92
 KenKen, 85, 92, 204
 left brain, 93–96
 Letter Scrambles, 94–96,
  100–102
 linking unrelated words, 9–10,
  37, 42, 45, 47
 mental exercise, 78–79
 N-back tests, 82–83
 Odd One Out exercises, 97, 103
 optimizing your brain game
  experience, 98
 Photo Recall exercises, 33–34
 popular, 92
 puzzles, 85
 recall practice, 204, 206,
  209–210, 212, 216, 218
 right brain, 93–96
 Sequence Recognition exercises,
  97–98, 103
 seven-word story exercises,
  224–225, 234–235
 Sorting Words exercises, 94, 100,
  232, 235

Straight Line Drawing exercises, 95, 101
Sudoku, 76, 85–86, 92, 99, 204
"Tip-of-the-Tongue" memory skills practice, 44, 49, 228, 235
Toothpick puzzles, 93, 100, 212, 214, 233
Trivial Pursuit, 92
video games, 82, 91–92
Visual Connecting exercises, 94–95, 97, 101–102
visual-spatial skills, 85, 88, 91–92, 94
websites, 237–238
whole brain, 94, 98
word generation exercises, 220, 230–231, 234, 235
word jumbles, 85–86, 100
word-pair recall, 224, 229, 232, 234
BrainBashers website, 237
Brain-derived neurotrophic factor (BDNF), 17–18, 128, 130, 148
Braingle website, 237
brainHQ website, 237
Breastfeeding, 81
Breathing exercises. See Meditation
Broca's area, 14–15, 87, 156
Broca's Area Language Center, 156

C

Caffeine
    effects of, 124–125
    in moderation, 126, 200
    sleep issues and, 69
    tea, 69, 117, 125–125
Calcium supplements, 189
Calcium, 189, 200
Calment, Jeanne, 24
Calories, 115–116
Cancer, 117, 119, 185–188
Carbohydrates, 115–116, 121–123, 200
Cardiovascular disease, 113, 143, 189
Centers for Disease Control and Prevention (CDC), 137–138

"Central obesity," 112
Cerebellum, 14–15, 87
Changing Words exercise, 93, 100
Chemical markers. See FDDNP; Glucose
Chest pain, 168
Chi energy, 71–72. See also Tai chi
Cholesterol
    apolipoprotein E (APOE) and, 17
    "bad" (LDL) cholesterol, 17, 112, 121, 178
    "good" (HDL) cholesterol, 112, 121
    statin drugs, 176, 178
Chronic traumatic encephalopathy (CTE), 138–139
ClinicalTrials.gov website, 241
Coconut oil, 119
Coenzyme Q10 supplements, 190
Cognitive behavioral therapy, 61–63
Cognitive intelligence. See IQ (intelligence quotient)
Concentration matching game, 82–83
Concussions, 5, 138
Confusion, 5, 53, 138, 175, 178, 182
Continuous partial attention, 68, 79
Corpus callosum, 11, 87–88
Cortisol, 21–22, 52–54, 62, 68, 155
Counting Squares exercise, 93, 100
Cousins, Norman, 166
Crossword puzzles, 44, 77, 85, 92, 204, 211
Crystallized intelligence, 81–82
CT scanning, 113
CTE. See Chronic traumatic encephalopathy
Curcumin, 190
Cycling, 138–139, 142

D

Dakim BrainFitness website, 91, 237
Dana Alliance for Brain Initiatives, 241
Dancing, 143

Dementia, 13–17, 57–58
   brain injury, 138–139
   diet and, 116, 120, 125
   dietary supplements and,
     190–193
   emotional disorders and, 57–58,
     61, 157
   exercise and, 127–129, 134
   Lewy bodies and, 182–183
   obesity and, 112, 115
   valium-induced, 182
   vascular dementia, 182–183
Dendrites, 152–153
Depression, 60–61
   nature vs. nurture in, 60
   sleep issues and, 65
   stress and, 53–54, 60–63, 73
   symptoms of, 60, 73
   treating. *See* Acupuncture;
     Cognitive behavioral therapy;
     Physical exercise; Relaxation
     techniques
Depression:;physiology of, 61
Deydroepiandrosterone (DHEA), 21,
   168, 185
DHA. *See* Docosahaxaednoic acid
DHEA. *See* Deydroepiandrosterone
Diabetes, 112–113
   body mass index and, 113
   glycemic index and, 123–124
   insulin, 114, 122–124, 145, 185, 188
   physical exercise and, 131, 141, 144
   stress and, 155
   symptoms of, 113
Diagnostic and Statistical Manual of
   Mental Disorders (DSM), 110–111
Diazepam (Valium), 182
Diet and nutrition, 105–126. *See also*
   Supplements; Obesity; Vitamins;
   Weight management; *specific*
   categories of food
     alcohol, 125–126. *See also*
       Alcohol consumption
     antioxidants. *See* Antioxidants

   brain inflammation, 118–120
   brain-healthy diet, 197
   caffeine, 124–125
   calorie restriction, 115–116
   fasting, 115–116
   fats. *See* Oils and fats
   fighting temptation, 107–108
   food addiction, 108–112
   fruits and vegetables, 23–24,
     116–117
   full-fat yogurt, 122
   ketogenic diet, 115–116
   low-carbohydrate/low-calorie
     diet, 115–116
   Mediterranean diet, 120–122
   mood and, 108–109
   nutritional habits, 105–107, 111,
     120
   portion control, 108, 111, 197
   protein, 121–123
   salt, 179
   snacks, 123–124, 199
   spices, 118
   sugar, 123–124. *See also* Sugar
Dietary Supplement and Health
   Education Act, 188
Divorce, 3, 15, 58, 108–109, 160
Docosahexaenoic acid (DHA), 119, 191
Doctors, 174–177, 180–182,
   186–187
Donepezil (Aricept), 173, 182–184
Dopamine, 19, 22, 111, 134, 167, 169
Dorsolateral region, 107
Double-blind, placebo-controlled
   clinical trials, 172, 190
Drugs and medications. *See also*
   Antioxidants; Supplements;
   Vitamins; specific drugs
     anti-inflammatory drugs, 67,
       179–180
     overreliance on, 180–182
     over-the-counter medicines,
       175, 181, 193. *See also* specific
       medicines

placebo effect, 119, 172–173, 178
to treat cognitive impairment,
182–185
DSM. *See* Diagnostic and Statistical
Manual of Mental Disorders

E

Edema, 186
Eicosapentaenoic acid (EPA), 191
Einstein, Albert, 11, 88
Elavil (amitriptyline), 185
Electrocardiograms, 176
Empathy, 61, 163–166
Endorphins, 21–22, 128
anti-inflammatory effects of, 67
elevated levels of, 69, 72, 136
as a natural analgesic, 134, 136
sexual activity and, 168
Enlarged prostate, 187
EPA. *See* Eicosapentaenoic acid
Estrogen, 185–187, 189
Executive functioning, 91–92, 129,
192
Exelon (rivastigmine), 182–183
Exercise. *See* Brain training; Physical
exercise
Eye contact, 70, 154, 156, 162, 208

F

Fasting, 115–116
Fats. *See* Oils and fats
FDDNP chemical marker, 13–14,
138–139, 183
Fight-or-flight response, 52
Finding Colors, 95, 101
Finicky Frank, 98, 103
Fish and seafood, 105–106, 119–121.
See also Omega-3 fatty acids
excess mercury, 120, 241
wild-caught vs. farmed, 119–120
The Flamingo (balance practice),
147–148, 211
FlaxSeed, 120, 126, 197
Fluid intelligence, 77, 81–82

FOCUS memory method, 32–36.
See also FRAME memory method;
Memory aids
memorizing unrelated words, 47,
209, 213, 214, 221, 227
memory places, 208
for names and faces, 35–36, 207,
227, 229, 230
for "tip-of-the-tongue" methods,
43–44, 48–49, 222, 228
for to-do lists, 42, 226–227
Folate (folic acid), 191
Food and Drug Administration
(FDA), 171–172
Forgetfulness. *See* Memory lapses
FRAME memory method, 32,
35–38. *See also* FRAME memory
method; Memory aids
memorizing unrelated words, 47,
206, 209, 213, 214, 215, 221, 227
memory places, 208
for names and faces, 35–36, 207,
227, 229, 230
for "tip-of-the-tongue" methods,
43–44, 48–49, 222, 228
for to-do lists, 42, 226–227
Frontal lobe, 11, 14–15, 36–37,
86–87, 154–156, 164–165
Functional MRI, 11, 19, 22, 36, 72,
89, 179

G

GABA (gamma amino butyric acid),
136
Galantamine (Razadyne), 182–183
Gallup Poll, 4, 116, 197
Gambling habits, 108–109
Games, 91–92. *See also* Brain training
Genetics, 15–19
apolipoprotein E (APOE), 16–19
brain-derived neurotrophic
factor (BDNF), 17–18, 128,
130, 148
identical twins, 15–16, 80

"smart genes," 78
TREM2 gene, 18
Germaphobia (mysophobia), 29
Gerontological Society of America,
    241
Ginkgo biloba, 188, 192
Glucose, 12–13, 119, 123–124
The Grey Labyrinth website, 238

H
Head trauma, 24, 36, 137–139
Headache, 5, 52, 54–55, 62, 138, 192
Healthcare, 171–193. *See also* Drugs
    and medications
        checklist, 175
        dietary supplements, 188–193.
            See also Antioxidants;
            Supplements; Vitamins
        doctors as partners, 173–175
        hormones for brain health,
            185–188. *See also* Hormones
        hypertension (high blood
            pressure), 178–179
        paternalistic healthcare model
            173–174
        physical illnesses and brain
            health, 175–178
The Healthy Brain Initiative, 241
Heart attacks, 21, 188–189
Heel-toe walk (balance exercise),
    223
HGH. *See* Human growth hormone
Hidden Proverb exercise, 95, 102
High blood pressure. *See*
    Hypertension
High glycemic index, 123
Highly superior autobiographical
    memory. *See* Photographic
    memory
Hippocampus, 14, 36–37, 61, 88–89,
    130, 168, 173
Hoarding, 29
Holocaust survivors, 58
Homocysteine, 191

Hormones, 185–188
    deydroepiandrosterone, 21, 168,
        185
    estrogen, 185–186, 189
    human growth hormone, 186
    progestogen, 186–187
    somatoliberin, 186
    testosterone, 186–188
Human growth hormone (HGH),
    186
Humor, 88, 166–167
Huperzine A, 192
Hydration, 197
Hypertension (high blood pressure),
    21, 54, 62, 106, 118, 141, 177–179,
    193
Hyperthymesia, *See* Photographic
    memory
Hypothalamus, 154
Hypothetical Country, 96–97, 102

I
Ibuprofen (Motrin, Advil), 179–180
Identical twins, 15–16, 80
Imipramine (Tofranil), 185
Immunoglobulin A antibody, 21, 168
Impulse control, 61, 113
Inflammation
    anti-inflammatory drugs, 67,
        179–180
    brain inflammation, 73, 118, 191
    sleep issues and, 65
Influenza, 175
Insomnia, 63–65, 182–183
Institute of Medicine, 189
Insula, 61, 155, 164–165
Insulin, 114, 122–124, 145, 185, 188
IQ (intelligence quotient), 80–83

J
Jigsaw Brain Breaks, 94, 96, 101, 100
Jigsaw puzzles, 75, 84, 92
*Journal of the American Medical
    Association Neurology*, 128

K

KenKen, 85, 92, 204
Ketogenic diets, 115–116
Ketone bodies, 116, 119

L

Late-life brain abnormalities. *See* Brain aging
Letter Scrambles, 94–96, 100–102
Lewy bodies, 182–183
Liver damage, 180, 187–188
"Love molecule," *See* Oxytocin
Lumosity website, 237
Lycopene, 117

M

Magnetic resonance imaging (MRI), 11–12, 22, 113, 155, 164–165
Marijuana, 20
Mayo Clinic, 139
Mazes, 78, 83–84, 92
MCI. *See* Mild cognitive impairment
Meal-Planning Brain Game, 114
Medical devices, 184
Medical imaging, 10–14. *See also* Functional magnetic resonance imaging; Magnetic resonance imaging; Positron-emission tomography
Meditation, 23, 59, 203–206. *See also* Stress; Stress management
breathing exercises, 205–206
mantra meditation, 221–222
mindfulness, 66–67
"on holiday," 212, 219
transcendental meditation, 66
Mediterranean diet, 120–122
Memantine (Namenda), 182–183
Memory, 27–49
age and, 2–3, 6–8
assessments of, 129–130, 202, 218, 233
cortisol and, 53
episodic memory, 43

errands and to-do lists, 42, 226–227
long term, 7, 29–30, 36, 213
memory habits, 40–42, 207, 209, 212, 214, 216, 219, 221, 224, 231
pencil-and-paper memory tests, 6, 12–13
photographic, 28–29
poor concentration and memory complaints, 60
prospective, 41–42, 205, 216, 222, 226
sensory, 29–31
short term, 7, 30, 37, 80, 82, 88–89, 218
visual, 7–7, 24
working memory, 7, 77, 82–83, 86
Memory aids. *See also* Brain training; FOCUS memory method; FRAME memory method
linking unrelated words, 9–10, 37, 42, 45, 47
memory places, 40–41, 49, 208, 222
Roman Room method, 44–45, 49, 220, 234
rote memorization vs., 9–10
story method, 213, 214, 216, 219, 224, 226
unhackable passwords, 46
Memory lapses, ix–x, 1–3. *See also* Brain aging; Tip-of-the-tongue moments
Memory places, 40–41, 49, 208, 222
Menopause, 186, 189
Mental exercises. *See* Brain training
Mental lapses. *See* Memory lapses
Metabolic syndrome, 65, 112–113
Metabolism, 121, 196
Mild cognitive impairment (MCI), 13–14

Alzheimer's disease and,
    183–184
brain injuries and, 139
caffeine, 125
defined, 139
depression and, 61
diet and, 121
human growth hormones and, 186
music and, 19
physical exercise and, 145
supplements and, 191–192
Misplacing objects. *See* Memory
    places
Mnemonics. *See* Memory aids
Monterey Bay Aquarium Seafood
    Watch, 120, 241
Motrin (ibuprofen), 179–180
MRI. *See* Magnetic resonance
    imaging (MRI) scans
Multitasking, 9, 68, 73, 79, 90–91
Music, 19–20, 38, 70, 81
Myelin, 5, 152–153
Mysophobia (fear of germs), 29

N
Namenda (memantine), 182–183
Naproxen (Aleve), 179, 180
National Center for Complementary
    and Alternative Medicine, 189, 242
National Council on Aging, 242
National Institute of Mental Health,
    242
National Institute of Neurological
    Disorders and Stroke, 242
National Institute on Aging, 242
N-back tests, 82–83
Neurodegeneration, 5, 61, 65–66,
    112, 117, 179
Neurogenesis (new nerve growth),
    24–25
Neurons, 5–6, 18–19, 84–87
Neuropsychological examinations, 6
Neurotransmitters
    acetylcholine, 182–183, 192

dopamine, 19, 22, 111, 134, 167,
    169
GABA (gamma amino butyric
    acid), 136
norepinephrine, 169
serotonin, 22, 60, 185
Nitric oxide, 178
Nonsteroidal anti-inflammatory
    drugs (NSAIDs), 180
Norepinephrine, 169
NSAIDs. *See* Nonsteroidal anti-
    inflammatory drugs (NSAIDs)
Nutrition. *See* Diet and nutrition
Nuts and *See*ds, 23–24, 117,
    119–123, 126, 197, 199–200

O
Obesity, 63, 106, 112–115. *See
    also* Diet and nutrition; Physical
    exercise; Weight management
    "central," 112
    definition of, 112
    dementia and, 115
    "obesity paradox," 115
    sugar and, 124
Obsessive-compulsive symptoms, 29
Odd One Out exercise, 97, 103
Oils and fats, 120. *See also*
    Cholesterol; Omega-3 fatty acids;
    Omega-6 fatty acids; Omega-9
    fatty acids
    coconut oil, 119
    essential, 118–119
    nonessential, 121
    olive oil, 114, 120–121, 198–199
    polyunsaturated fatty acids
        (PUFAs), 119
    saturated fat, 119
Omega-3 fatty acids, 23–24,
    118–120, 191–193
    docosahexaenoic acid (DHA),
        119, 191
    eicosapentaenoic acid (EPA), 191
    supplements, 191–192

Omega-6 fatty acids, 119–120, 197
Omega-9 fatty acids, 121
"On holiday" meditation, 212, 219
Osteoporosis, 144, 189
Overeaters Anonymous 12-step program, 111
Over-the-counter medicines, 175, 181, 193. *See also* specific medicines
Oxidation, 116, 197. *See also* Antioxidants
Oxytocin, 152, 155, 168–169

P

Pain
    acupuncture, 71–72
    back pain, 22, 62–63, 137
    chest, 168
    chronic pain, 54, 63, 67
    cognitive behavioral therapy and, 63
    dysfunctional relationships and, 63
Pancreas, 123
Parietal lobe, 14–15, 87
Parkinson's disease, 125
PedagoNet website, 237
Peg method, 46–47, 49
PET. *See* Positron-emission tomography
Pew Research Internet Project, 174
Phosphatidylserine, 192–193
Photo Recall exercises, 33–34
Photographic memory, 28–29
Physical exercise, 127–150
    accessory-free isometrics, 145
    aerobic conditioning, 127
    aerobic fitness, 141–144. *See also* Aerobic fitness
    aging and, 128–129
    baseline fitness, 132–133, 200
    brain health and, 129–132
    brain-protective effects of, 133–134
    chair workout, 144

competitive sports, 143
complete fitness program, 140–141
core muscle groups, 148
daily goal, 201
depression and, 22
endorphins and, 22
finding an exercise buddy or group, 142
head trauma or brain injury, 137–140
heart-rate monitors, 141
isolation exercises with, 147
making it fun, 132–136
minimizing pain and, 136–137
mood-lifting effect of e, 128
resistance band, 146
resistance exercises, 144
risk for injury, 131
safer sports alternatives, 140
sense of balance, 147–150. *See also* Balance work
short-term cognitive benefits of, 128
side bends, 202–203
split routines, 145–146
strength training, 144–147. *See also* Strength training
swimming, 142–143
tips to make exercise fun, 134
weight training, 145
Physical therapy, 132, 137
Phytonutrients, 117
Pilates, 148
Pneumonia, 175
Polyunsaturated fatty acids (PUFAs), 119
Pomegranates, 116–117, 190
Portion control, 108, 111, 197
Positron-emission tomography (PET), 11–14, 18, 28, 65, 138–139
    FDDNP chemical marker, 13–14, 138–139, 183
Post-traumatic stress disorder (PTSD), 54, 59–60, 62

Prednisone, 182
Preferred hand, 87–88, 204, 218, 232
Prefrontal cortex, 107, 167
Premarin, 186
Processed foods, 106, 197
Progestogen, 186–187
Prosphatidylserine, 192–193
Prostate cancer, 187–188
Prozac, 185
Psychodynamic therapy, 60–61
PTSD. *See* Post-traumatic stress
    disorder
PUFAs. *See* Polyunsaturated fatty
    acids (PUFAs)

R
Rapid eye movement (REM) sleep, 64
Razadyne (galantamine), 182–183
Rebound REM (rapid eye
    movement), 64
Recall
    games to practice, 204, 206,
        209–210, 212, 216, 218
    Photo Recall exercises, 33–34
    story, 222–223, 226
    word-pair, 224, 229, 232, 234
Relaxation techniques, 3, 30, 64, 70,
    203. *See also* Meditation; Tai chi;
    Yoga
    sleep issues and, 70–71. *See also*
        Sleep issues
Reticular formation, 84
Rivastigmine (Exelon), 182–183
Roman Room method, 44–45, 49,
    220, 234
Rote memorization, 9–10
Russian folk dance (conditioning
    exercise), 203

S
Salt, 118, 179
Scrabble, 76, 91–92
Selective serotonin reuptake
    inhibitors (SSRIs), 185

Self-assessment, 55
Self-chats, 70
Self-confidence, 73
Self-regulation, 106–107
"Senior moments." *See* Memory slips
SeniorNet, 242
Sense of balance. *See* Balance
    training
Sensorimotor strip, 14–15, 156
Sensory memories, 29–31
Sequence Recognition exercises,
    97–98, 103
Serotonin, 22, 60, 185
Seven-word story exercises,
    224–225, 234–235
Sexual activity
    daily, 20–21
    dehydroepiandrosterone
        (DHEA), 21, 168, 185
    immune system and, 21
    libido, 185, 187
Sharp Brains website, 238
Singh, Fauja, 135
Sleep issues
    age and need for, 69
    amyloid proteins and, 65
    apnea, 187
    caffeine and, 69
    inflammation and, 65
    insomnia, 63–65, 182–183
    naps, 69
    rebound REM, 64
    relaxation techniques, 70–71.
        See also Relaxation techniques
    sleep deprivation, 63–65
    sleep strategies, 69–71
    stress and, 63–65, 69–71
"Smart drugs," 171–172
"Smart genes," 78
Snacks, 123–124, 199
Social interactions, 151–170
    attentive listening, 165
    divorce, 3, 15, 58, 108–109, 160
    empathy and, 163–166

expressing understanding, 165
fine-tuning your listening skills, 162
good habits, 160–163
good vs. not-so-good friends, 159
healthy relationships for better brain health, 170
importance of face-to-face conversations, 170
laughter and, 166–167
oxytocin and, 152. *See also* Oxytocin
rejection and brain activity, 155
sex and love, 167–169. *See also* Sexual activity
social neuroscience, 153–155
spending time with family and friends, 155–157
support systems, 157–160
talking and listening, 208
technology and, 169–170
toxic relationships, 162–163
videoconferencing, 170
Somatoliberin, 186
Somatosensory cortex, 155
Sorting Words exercises, 94, 100, 232, 235
Spinal cord, 84
SSRIs. *See* Selective serotonin reuptake inhibitors
Stanford-Binet test, 80
Story recall, 222–223, 226
Straight Line Drawing exercises, 95, 101
Strength training, 144–147. *See also* Physical exercise
bicep curls, 146, 214
dumbbells and weight-lifting machines, 144
free weights, 146
isolation exercises with resistance bands, 146
isometric, 145

mood and, 145
pull-down with squats, 148
recommendations for older adults, 146
upper body pull-down (strength training), 146, 221
Stress management, 64, 65–74. *See also* Physical exercise; Relaxation techniques
cutting back on multitasking, 68
getting organized, 71
laughter, 68–69
optimism and positive attitudes, 72–73
*See*king help, 73–74
self-chats, 70
sexual activity and, 167–168
skills, 54–55
sleep and, 63–65, 69–71
Stress, 3, 51–74
acute vs. chronic, 52–53
assessing, 54–56
causes of, 54
dementia risk and, 58
depression and, 53–54, 60–63, 73
effects of, 21–22, 53, 55–59
fight-or-flight response, 52
oxidative stress attacks, 189
panic attacks, 62
physical symptoms of, 53–54
reduction, 64, 65–74. *See also* Stress management
Strokes, 11, 177–179
defined, 179
mini-strokes, 177–178
risk of, 121
Subdural hematomas, 188
Sudoku, 76, 85–86, 92, 99, 204
Sugar
glucose, 12–13, 119, 123–124
blood sugar, 112, 155, 122–123, 144, 185. *See also* Diabetes
refined, 197
Suicide, 60

Supplements, 188–193. *See also* Antioxidants; Drugs and medications; Vitamins
  acetyl-l-carnitine supplements, 190
  calcium, 189
  Coenzyme Q10, 190
  dementia and, 190–193
  ginkgo biloba, 188, 192
  mild cognitive impairment and, 191–192
  omega-3 fatty acids, 191–192
  pomegranate capsules, 190
Synapses, 5, 153
Syvum website, 238

T

Tai chi, 67, 73, 139, 148
Talk therapy. *See* Cognitive behavioral therapy
tDCS. *See* Transcranial direct current stimulation
Tea, 69, 117, 125–125
Technology
  effect on the brain, 79, 89
  social interactions and, 169–170
  unhackable passwords, 46
Temporal lobe, 14–15, 59, 72, 87–89, 156, 163
Temporal mandibular joint (TMJ) syndromes, 62
Testosterone, 186–188
Tetrahydrocannabinol (THC), 20
THC. *See* Tetrahydrocannabinol
Thyroid imbalance, 23, 175, 181–182
TIAs. *See* Transient ischemic attacks
Tip-of-the-tongue moments, 42–44, 48–49, 222, 228
  memory skills practice, 44, 49, 228, 235
  reducing frequency of, 43–44
TMJ. *See* Temporal mandibular joint (TMJ) syndromes
TOFI (thin outside, fat inside), 113
Tofranil (imipramine), 185

Toothpick puzzles, 93, 100, 212, 214, 233
Touch therapy. *See* Acupressure
Transcendental meditation, 66
Transcranial direct current stimulation (tDCS), 184
Transdermal patches, 183
Transient ischemic attacks (TIAs), 177–178
TREM2 gene, 18
Tricky Riddles website, 238
Triglycerides, 112
Tumors, 11. *See also* Cancer
Turmeric. *See* Curcumin
Twisting boxer (conditioning exercise), 213–214
Tylenol (acetaminophen), 175–176, 180

U

UCLA Longevity Center, 243
Ulcerative colitis, 21
The Ultimate Puzzle Site website, 238
University of South Florida Health Byrd Alzheimer's Institute, 119, 125
Upper body pull-down (strength training), 146, 221
Urinary tract infection, 175
US Dept. of Veterans Affairs, 243
US Preventive Services Task Force, 189

V

Valium (diazepam), 182
Vascular dementia, 182–183
Ventromedial cortex, 107
Video games, 8–9, 76, 79–80, 82, 91–92
Videoconferencing, 170
Virginia Cognitive Aging Project, 43
Visual aids, 38
Visual Connecting exercises, 94–95, 97, 101–102
Visual cortex, 14–15, 87, 156

Visual-spatial skills, 10
    games, 85, 88, 91–92, 94
Vitamins. *See also* Supplements
    Vitamin A, 188
    Vitamin B, 191, 200
    Vitamin B6, 191
    Vitamin C, 190
    Vitamin D, 188, 191
    Vitamin E, 188–190
    Vitamin K, 188

W
WAIS. *See* Wechsler Adult
    Intelligence Scale
Walking, 141–142
    baseline fitness and, 132–135
    creativity and, 142
    diabetes and, 131
    as part of a fitness program, 129,
        204
    risk for injury and, 141–142, 201
    sleep issues and, 69

Wechsler Adult Intelligence Scale
    (WAIS), 80
Weight loss (unexplained), 60, 113,
    115
Weight management. *See also* Diet
    and nutrition; Obesity
    bariatric surgery, 114
    compulsiveness, 109
    Overeaters Anonymous 12-step
        program, 111
    portion control, 108, 111, 197
    unusual weight loss, 60, 113, 115
White matter, 121, 153
Women's Health Initiative, 186
World Health Organization, 112, 116

Y
Yahoo! Games website, 238
Yoga, 67, 73, 135–136, 149–150

Z
Zoloft, 185